Lenses, Spectacles, Eyeglasses, and Contacts

Lenses, Spectacles, Eyeglasses, and Contacts

The Story of Vision Aids

Alberta Kelley

ELSEVIER/NELSON BOOKS
New York

Library of Congress Cataloging in Publication Data

Kelley, Alberta.
Lenses, spectacles, eyeglasses, and contacts.

Bibliography: p. 92
Includes index.
SUMMARY: Presents a history of vision aids from ancient times to the present and discusses the medical care offered by ophthalmologists, optometrists, and opticians, and what new developments can be expected in the future.
1. Ophthalmic lenses—Juvenile literature. 2. Eyeglasses—Juvenile literature. 3. Contact lenses—Juvenile literature. [1. Eyeglasses. 2. Contact lenses] I. Title.
RE976.K44 617.7'52 78-14827
ISBN 0-525-66617-6

Published in the United States by Elsevier/Nelson Books, a division of Elsevier-Dutton Publishing Company, Inc., New York. Published simultaneously in Don Mills, Ontario, by Thomas Nelson and Sons (Canada) Limited.

Printed in the U.S.A. First Edition

10 9 8 7 6 5 4 3 2

For Tom, Ben, and Mary

Acknowledgments

Several persons contributed to my research for this book. For their patience and assistance, my thanks to Lawrence O. Aasen, Executive Secretary, Better Vision Institute; to Dr. Alden Haffner, President, and staff members, of the New York State College of Optometry; and to William Madden of Berks Optical Company and I. Martin Laurel. Other individuals—ophthalmologists, optometrists, and librarians—were extremely helpful.

For her editorial assistance and unfailing encouragement, I am deeply indebted to Jean Mercier.

Contents

Introduction

Recently, in a local optician's fitting room, a customer sat nervously waiting for her eyeglasses to be adjusted. Her pronounced frown and squint indicated that, without a vision aid, she was extremely nearsighted. When the optician had completed the adjustment and placed her eyeglasses in position, the woman's face was instantly transformed. The frown disappeared, her facial muscles relaxed, her eyes became naturally wider. "It's wonderful to see again," she commented.

Most spectacle wearers can recall the relief they felt when first fitted with glasses to help them read comfortably or see distant objects. It is estimated that Americans spend more than five billion dollars annually on this eye care. Almost one hundred million of us wear eyeglasses or contact lenses. Techniques to correct vision defects also include surgery and vision training.

The search for ways to help the visually impaired has been a dramatic one, and a host of scientists, doctors, and other professionals have been a part of it. Their story extends from ancient times to the present. Who were they? How did they work their wonders? What new developments can be expected in the ophthalmic field in the future? This book considers these questions in an overview of eye care.

1

Beginnings

Today's sophisticated, decorative eyeglasses are a far cry from the round piece of crude quartz through which the ancients peered. Designed to express the wearer's personality and to conform to current fashion, they run the gamut from saucer shapes, big as headlights, to less conspicuous, rimless spectacles. Sometimes glasses lend the wearer a look of distinction. The mousy clerk looks more impressive, almost like an executive, behind his heavy rimmed specs. A vacant, nondescript face miraculously assumes a thoughtful, scholarly expression with glasses. And, as many actors know, contact lenses containing a color component can change the color of the eye. As early as 1940, blue-eyed Walter Hampden became a brown-eyed Indian in the film *Northwest Mounted Police.* Sir Lawrence Olivier is said to have a number of pairs of contacts in various colors to suit different characters.

More importantly, today's eyeglasses are expertly designed to correct the wearer's vision defects. They are the result of nine centuries of scientific search and discovery.

We find it difficult now to imagine life without prescription eyeglasses, but that is how people lived for centuries. They had to rely upon simple magnification, or nothing.

The treatments offered to patients with sight defects in the Dark Ages sound like black magic to us today. For strengthening weak sight one medical treatise recommended hanging a cow's eye from the neck of the afflicted. For a man with a pain in the eye, it was prescribed "to tie in unwrought flax as many knots as there are letters in his name, pronouncing them as you go, and tie it around his neck." But for a truly bizarre approach nothing tops this formula: ". . . catch a fox alive, cut his tongue out; let him go; dry his tongue and tie it up in a red rag and hang it round the man's neck." A few incantations accompanied this procedure.

Master John of Arden enthusiastically recommended a most original concoction in a 1377 book:

> For watery eyes, if the patient be aged and decrepit, this ointment provides the best cure. . . . Use a basin of brass, well greased with fresh butter, and let it stand overnight; in the morning let the basin be inverted upon a pot or dish in which is the sour urine of a man, warmed that it may

> receive the most urine. Let the butter be melted and when cool take down the basin and thus let it stand for a whole day; afterward let the butter be scraped out (it will appear green) and mix with it a little fat of a capon liquefied by the sun's heat or a fire and store it up in a waxed vessel. Let the eyelid be well anointed. . . . This medicine was highly beneficial to my own eyes studying and writing until the seventieth year of my age. . . . I . . . the least of surgeons [he concludes, poignantly] wrote this little book painfully with my own hand at London in the first year of King Richard the Second. . . .

Dr. Walter Bayley, physician to Elizabeth I, wrote what is believed to be the first book on eyesight in English. His recommendations included the suggestion that our vision may be affected by the position in which we sleep. "Best to begin the sleep upon the right side and then turn on the left side," he advises. He cautions against sleeping "in a chamber or any place where the moon shines."

Later, piercing the ears was thought to benefit weak eyesight.

The story of how spectacles were developed is a tribute to the perseverance of scientists and a classic example of the incredibly slow evolution of an important idea. In the eleventh century, Alhazen, an Arabian scientist, was struggling to understand and define vision. He concluded that "the ideas of external objects are conveyed by the optic nerves to the brain." He also believed that rays of light proceed from a visible object to the eye of the observer.

At a time when anatomical knowledge was severely limited, this was revolutionary thinking. It reversed Pythagoras's sixth-century B.C. theory that a set of rays emerged from the eye and struck objects so that information was passed back by the lens to the brain. Euclid, too, held this theory two centuries later, but Aristotle, at about the same time, quite reasonably pointed out that if this

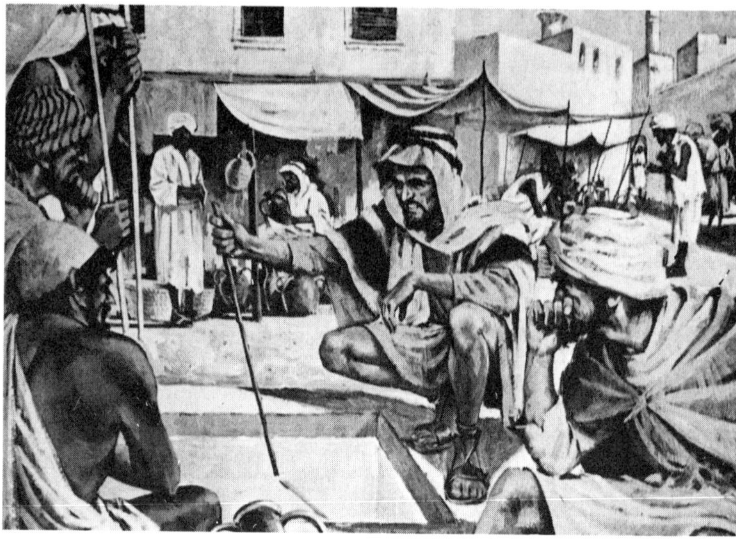

An artist's conception of Alhazen demonstrating the refraction of light
Hilco, a Division of the Hilsinger Corporation

were true, vision should be as good at night as in the day. Furthermore, said Aristotle (less accurately), the lens of the eye did not exist until a coagulation formed after death.

And so it went, with the ball bouncing back and forth, while more and more attention was given to the phenomenon of magnification: first as the Greeks knew it, through water-filled spheres, then through quartz or other natural formations. Nero is said to have used an emerald ring to aid his vision.

A Polish scientist, Vitello, who preceded Isaac Newton, author of the impressive *Optiks* (1704), by several hundred years, was the first European to write a book on optics. In the thirteenth century, Vitello reported on lenses: "The convex surface brings the rays [of light] together and the concave produces divergence."

Knowledge about light rays and refraction was now emerging in many places. The Islamic world had been conducting experiments in magnification with glass spheres since A.D. 1000. The Chinese had magnifying glasses of rock crystal and dark glasses of smoky quartz by the twelfth century. Marco Polo reported seeing spectacles in China at the end of the thirteenth century.

Ten years after Vitello's *Treatise on Optics* (1270), John Peckham, archbishop of Canterbury, wrote *Prospectiva Communis*, which summarized contemporary optical knowledge. Leonardo da Vinci expanded on Peckham's views and wrote a book which, translated, is called *An Introduction to Perspective, That Is to Say to the Function of the Eye*. Leonardo discovered that the retina was the essential organ of vision, and left drawings of proposed lens-grinding machines among his amazingly varied scientific inquiries.

In England, in 1257, Friar Roger Bacon was imprisoned by his own order, the Franciscans, for his unorthodox ideas. His scientific daring continued to cause so much suspicion and fear that he was confined again at the end of his life (1278–1292). One of his "crimes" was writing *Opus Majus* (1268). He declared,

> If anyone examine letters or other minute objects through the medium of crystal or glass or other transparent substance, if it be shaped like the lesser segment of a sphere, with the convex side towards the eye, he will see the letters far better and they will seem larger. . . . For this reason such an instrument is useful to all persons and to those with weak eyes, for they can see any letter, however small, if magnified enough."

During his first imprisonment, Bacon sent Pope Clement IV, a secret admirer, magnifying lenses for reading. Perhaps it was from Bacon's experiments that thirteenth-century monks, bending over their illuminated manuscripts, hit upon the idea of spectacles. Anyway, Bacon shares the honors for inventing them with an unknown Chinese, a couple of Italians, and a German or two.

The first glasses in Italy were attributed by some to Alessandro di Spina of Florence, but Salvino d'Armato

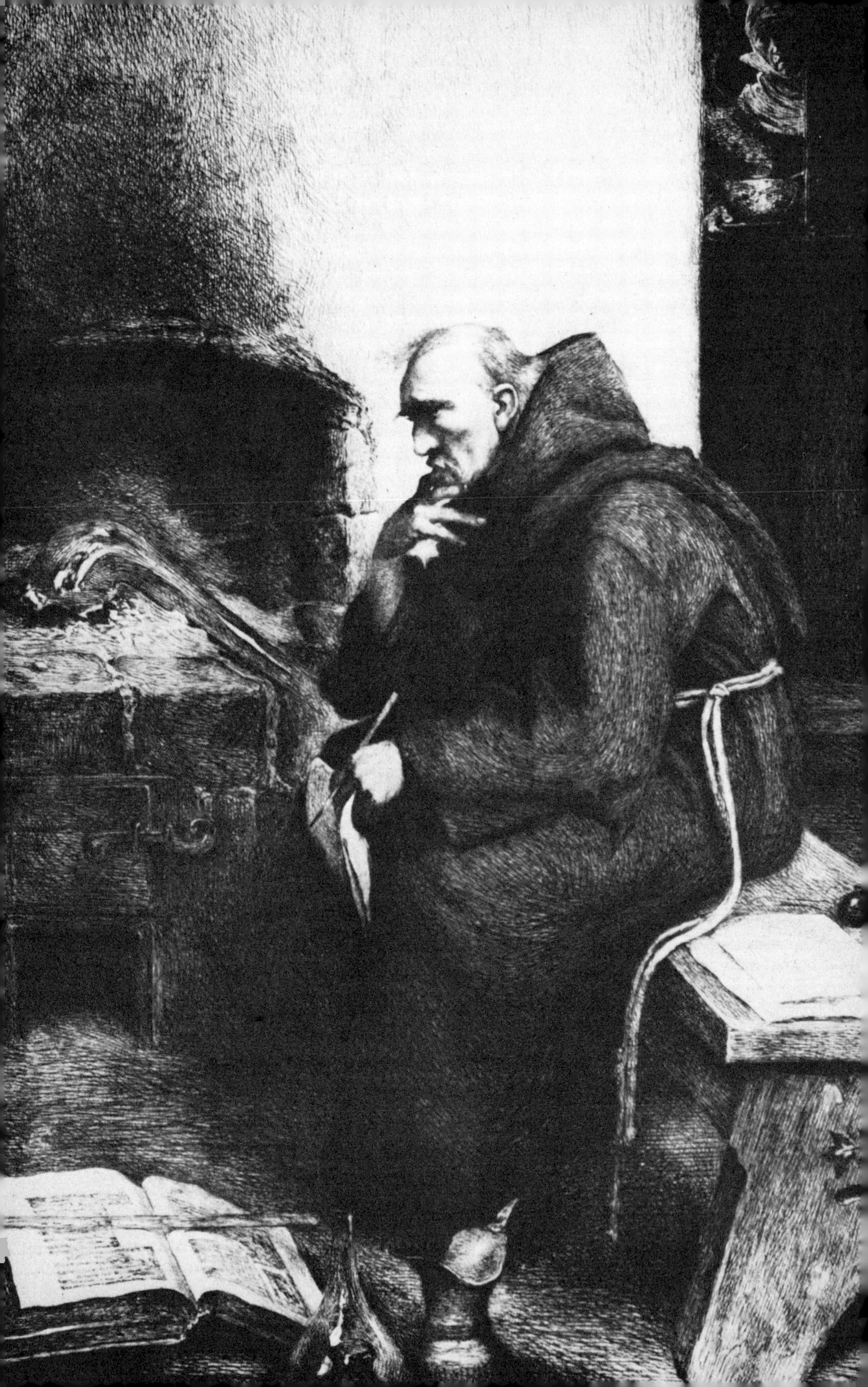

also comes into the picture at the beginning of the fourteenth century. The epitaph on his tombstone in Florence reads, "Here lies Salvino d'Armato of the Armati of Florence. Inventor of spectacles. God pardon him his sins. A.D. 1317." The last sentence wasn't just a conventional plea for forgiveness. At that time, wearing spectacles was considered the height of sinfulness.

We can place the first use of spectacles fairly within a hundred-year span. Chaucer, in "The Wife's Tale" (1386), wrote:

Povert a spectakel is, as thinkith me
Thurgh which he may his verray frendes se.

And Sandra di Popozo, author in 1289 of *Traite di conduite de la famille*, described the experience of many modern elderly people when he said, "I am so debilitated by age that without the glasses known as spectacles, I would no longer be able to read or write. These have recently been invented for the benefit of poor old people whose sight has become weak." Today the "poor old people" have ceased to marvel, and pretty much take their glasses for granted. But to Popozo, they were a sight-saving miracle.

Although the development of spectacles crept along, the farsighted were using them widely by the fifteenth century. Several centuries more had to pass, however, before someone solved the problem of keeping glasses securely on the nose!

Opposite. Etching of Friar Roger Bacon by Wm. H. W. Bicknell, after a painting by Howard Pyle.
Prints Division, The New York Public Library, Astor, Lenox and Tilden Foundations

2

Refraction

Until the seventeenth century vision defects were corrected by trial and error. Johannes Kepler, a German astronomer, defined myopia (nearsightedness) in 1604. It was the first time an eye defect was given a name. Hyperopia (farsightedness) was defined in the mid-1800's by the Dutch ophthalmologist, Frans Cornelis Donders, author of the still unrefuted text, *On the Anomalies of Accommodation and Refraction of the Eye* (1864). In between these two events, in 1793, we find the English physicist Thomas Young defining astigmatism, a defect resulting from irregularities in the surface of the lens or cornea. Sir George Airy, an English astronomer who suffered from astigmatism, invented the cylindrical lens that corrects the defect in 1827.

These definitions probably followed a period when diagnoses and prescriptions were already being given freely through educated guesswork. They were the culmination, in other words, of a long, long stretch of scientific activity.

A knowledge of how the eye functions is essential to understanding these discoveries. The miracle of sight is still a mystery today, but it has yielded a few of its secrets. Probably the most important discovery was the law of refraction, which Willebrord Snell, a Dutchman, worked out in the early seventeenth century.

The eye is a sphere composed of watery substance (aqueous humor) in front and a sticky viscous substance (vitreous humor) at it's back. The cornea, a tough, transparent layer covering the pupil, acts as a single refracting surface. It bends incoming light rays so that they intersect and form an image on the retina, which is located on the rear inner surface of the sphere. As in a camera, the retina receives an upside-down image, which is reversed by the brain.

The cornea provides about four fifths of the eye's refractive power; the rest is supplied by the eye's lens, which is suspended behind the pupil. If the dimensions of the eye or the curvature of the cornea or lens prevent light rays from focusing exactly on the retina, vision will be blurred. Hence, the defects we call nearsightedness (myopia), farsightedness (hyperopia), astigmatism, or presbyopia, depending on the symptoms, will occur.

A measure of the refraction of the eye determines the point where light rays are focused. If that point falls short

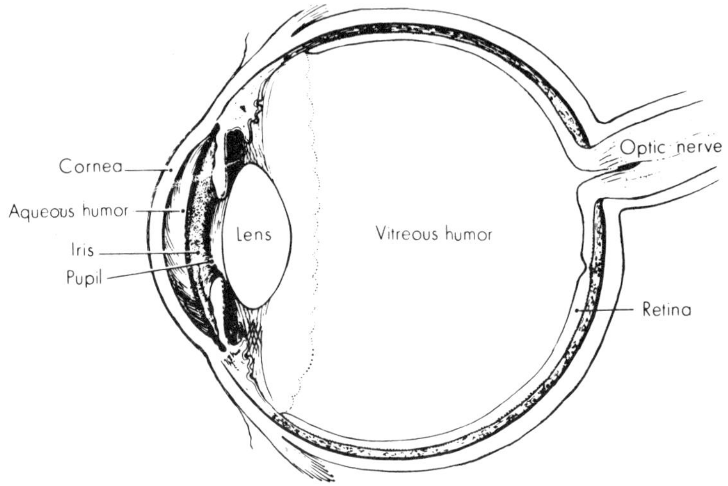

The eye *Better Vision Institute, Inc.*

How vision works *Better Vision Institute, Inc.*

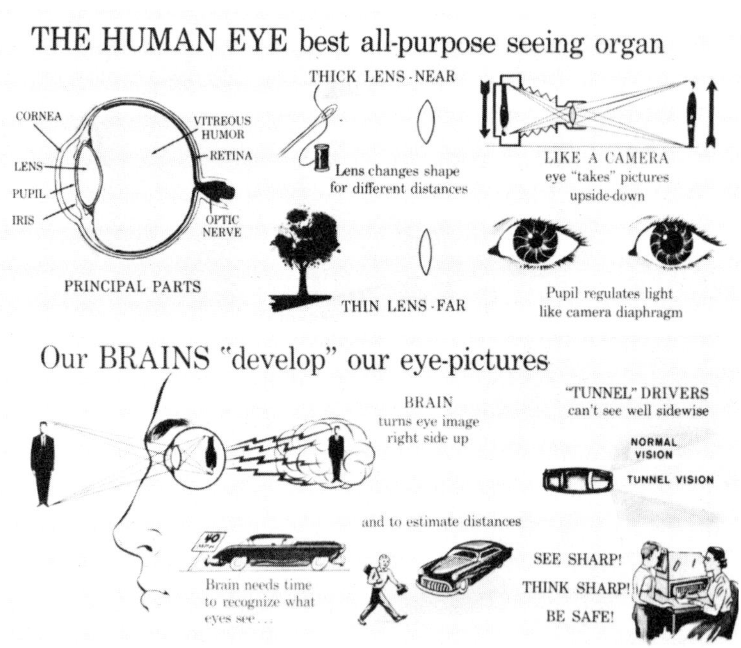

of, or extends beyond, the retina, corrective lenses are needed.

Snell's law of refraction—an important link in the chain of optical-glass development—remained unpublished until René Descartes reported it eleven years after Snell's death in 1626.

What exactly occurs in the vision process to cause imperfections?

The myopic eye focuses the light rays in front of the retina because the distance from the cornea and lens to the back of the eye is too great for the eye's refractive power. Without corrective glasses a blurred image results.

The direct opposite of myopia is hyperopia, in which the eye focuses light rays at a greater distance than exists from cornea and lens to retina. Although the hyperopic eye can see well at a distance, vision aid is necessary for reading, especially as a person gets older and develops presbyopia, a form of farsightedness caused by the loss of flexibility in the lens of the eye.

Astigmatism, a common defect, is due to an irregularity in the cornea's shape or an uneven curvature of the eye's lens. When this condition exists, the image on the retina is warped. If eyeglasses are recommended to correct astigmatism, they will have a cylindric lens like the one Sir George Airy invented. An astigmatic eye can also be myopic or hyperopic.

Two eye problems of a different nature, one of which is not amenable to correction by eyeglasses, are strabismus and color blindness.

Authorities tell us that three million Americans suffer from strabismus, which causes amblyopia, or lazy eye. What happens here is related to a focusing deficiency in which each eye transmits a different image. The visual cortex suppresses one of the two images. Hence, one eye develops, while the other gradually becomes incapable of vision. Strabismus may be hereditary, or it may be caused

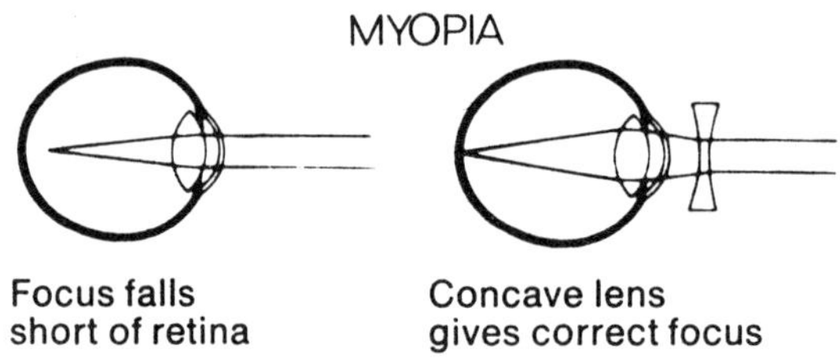

Myopia *Better Vision Institute, Inc.*

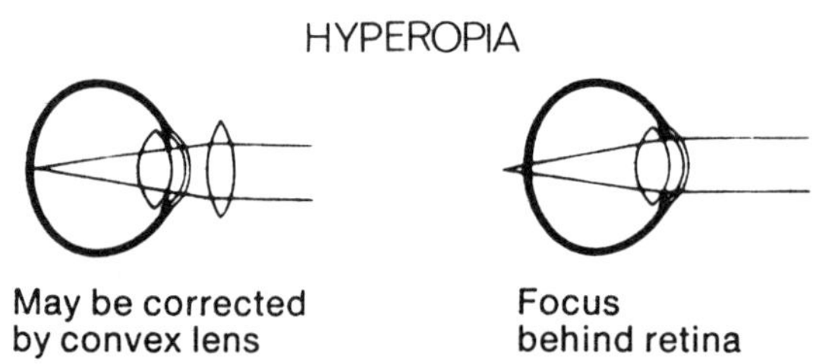

Hyperopia *Better Vision Institute, Inc.*

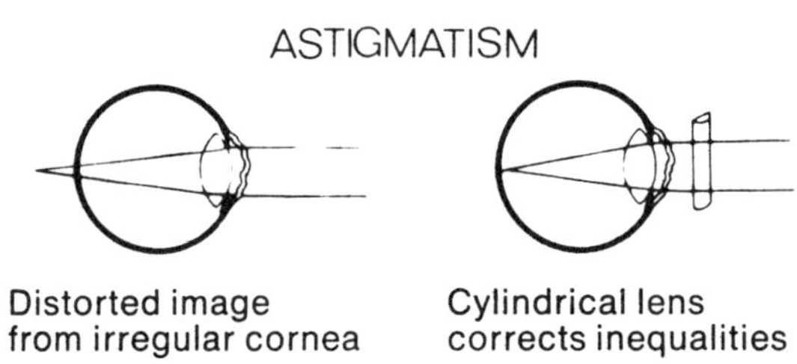

Astigmatism *Better Vision Institute, Inc.*

by an uneven development of the extraocular muscles, or by a deviation in the visual control center. If the normal eye is covered, the undeveloped one may be strengthened and regain almost normal sight, especially in children. But the underlying cause for the defect must be traced if both eyes are to remain normally sighted.

There are several variations of strabismus. In convergent strabismus one eye deviates inward; in divergent strabismus the affected eye drifts outward, or up, or down. Thus we have such terms as *cross-eyed, walleyed, squint.* Although vision therapy and/or eyeglasses may correct the problem, surgery is often recommended.

Eyeglasses may help strabismus, but "Daltonism" is an eye defect that no lens can completely correct. John Dalton (1766–1844), an Englishman, lived with his parents in a thatched cottage in Cumberland. He stumbled upon his color blindness when he bought his mother a pair of bright-red hose which he thought were dark blue, or so the story goes. Dalton, a chemist and physicist, had a scientist's interest in his defect. He studied it and, in 1794, published the first detailed description of "Daltonism."

Color blindness is believed to be caused by a deficiency in the eye's "receivers." This is part of the vision process that is still unknown, but we know that transmission from the retina to the brain is achieved by rod-shaped cells that "see" black and white, and by cone-shaped cells that "see" colors. These cells activate electrical signals sent to the brain's visual cortex.

Color blindness is hereditary. It rarely involves totally colorless sight (when that occurs it is called monochromasy), but is a deficiency in seeing colors. Women carry and transmit the abnormality, but less than one percent of all American and European women have the problem themselves. These few usually have both a color-blind father and a carrier mother. Tinted lenses will sometimes help color-blind persons distinguish different hues.

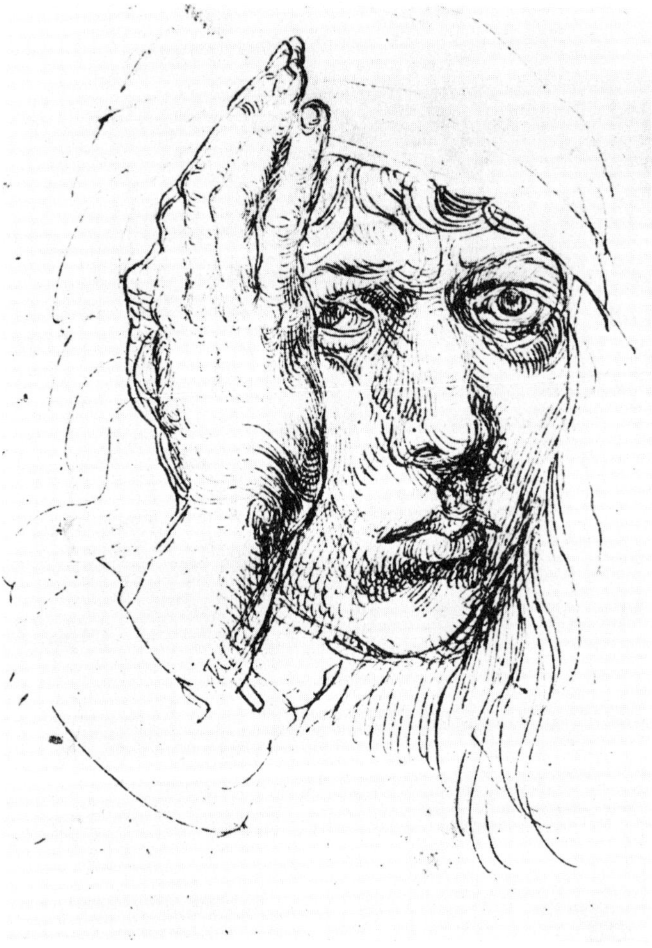

Self-portrait, Albrecht Dürer

The oldest painting showing spectacles is a portrait of Hugh of Provence, created by Tommaso da Modena in 1352. Hugh had died a century earlier, but the artist added the spectacles as a token of respect. Saint Paul was portrayed the same way in an illustrated manuscript done in 1380, as were Moses, in 1452, and Saint Peter, in a painting done around 1485. In 1517, Raphael painted Pope Leo X wearing spectacles containing concave lenses for myopia (the ones Vitello described).

An example that tops them all is found in a panel of a sculpture by Nicola Pisano (1225–1280) on the marble pulpit of the baptistery at Pisa. The sculptor depicted the infant Jesus wearing round spectacles with heavy, dark frames.

The relationship of vision defects to art is a fascinating study because of what some specialists think certain paintings may reveal about the eyesight of the artists themselves. According to the experts, El Greco and Holbein the Younger may have suffered from astigmatism. If one views their paintings through corrective cylindrical lenses, one finds that the characteristic distortion disappears. But, alas, the normalizing lenses also sacrifice the individuality that distinguishes the work of these artists. An English clergyman once observed, "The newly invented optick glasses are immoral, since they pervert the natural sight, and make things appear in an unnatural and false light." Of course spectacles were intended to do just the opposite. Their absence made each person a captive of his own particular defect. However, for a few artists with slight astigmatism, that was not necessarily a bad thing.

Nearsightedness and farsightedness, according to the experts, have had a direct influence on the color that predominates in an artist's work. The myope sees reds better, the hyperope is better equipped to see blues. Renoir is cited as an example of a myope fascinated with reds. The Chinese and Japanese are predominantly myopic, and it is presumed that their preference for reds is a result of their nearsightedness.

Presbyopia, experts believe, may account for the increasing "fuzziness" of paintings by long-lived artists such as Rembrandt and Titian. This is an adventurous speculation, and since the artists' professional growth and individual conceptions can never be separated from their visual acuity, the assumption must remain inconclusive.

Dürer has been named as an example of an artist with strabismus, a divergent squint in his case. His self-portrait of 1491 depicts him with right hand raised, warding off a confusing second image seen by the divergent eye.

El Greco's saints, as they look heavenward, also seem to have diverging eyes, and in his portrait of St. Luke, done in 1604, thought by many to be a self-portrait, the impression of strabismus is obvious.

Experts have diagnosed the maddening headaches described by Van Gogh as a symptom of glaucoma. Their diagnosis seems to be confirmed by the paintings in which he depicts lights and the sun with surrounding halos, an aberration typical of glaucoma.

Theorists have speculated on the possible relationship between eye strength and reading and writing customs. In Western countries, the right eye is usually dominant, and we read and write from left to right. In the East, where the left eye is believed to be the dominant one, people often read and write from right to left.

But intriguing as these digressions may be, they have led us away from the history of eyeglasses, which is more factual and equally engrossing.

3

Eye Examinations

Two men especially come to mind in any discussion of eye examinations. In 1863 Hermann Snellen introduced the familiar chart that bears his name and which is still the sine qua non of eye examinations. The term 20/20 vision simply means that at a distance of 20 feet the examinee can read a certain line on the chart.

Snellen was a pupil of fellow countryman Frans Donders, who is called the "Father of Modern Refraction." You may recall that Donders defined farsightedness and wrote

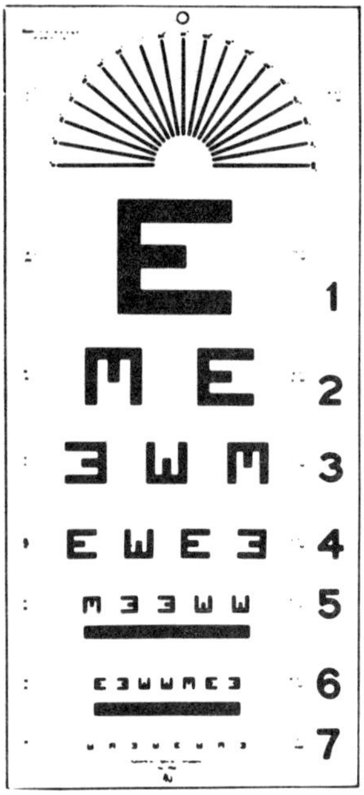

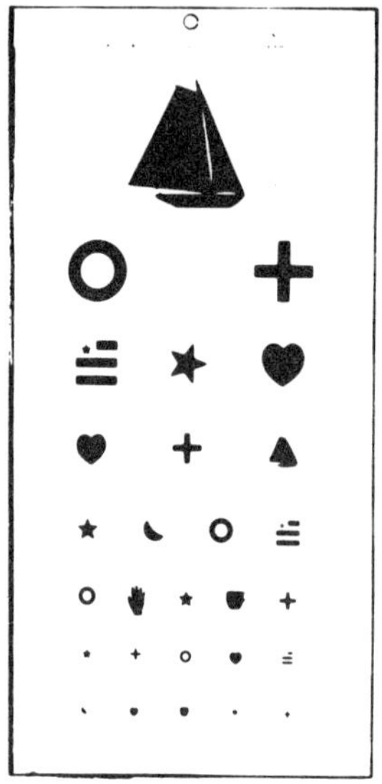

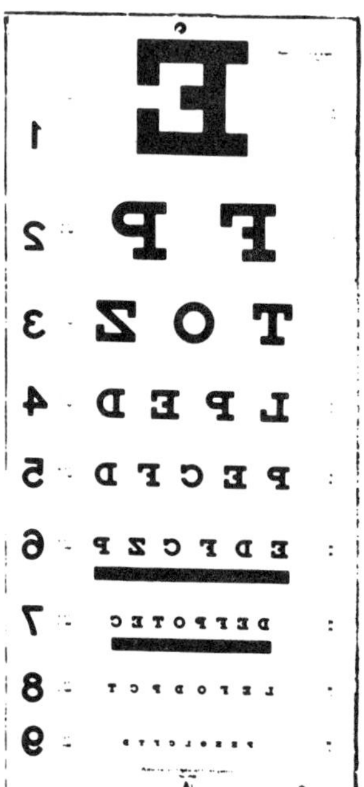

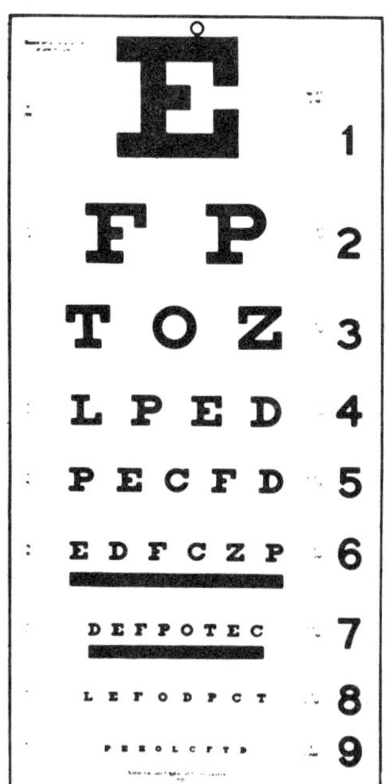
E 1
F P 2
T O Z 3
L P E D 4
P E C F D 5
E D F C Z P 6
D E F P O T E C 7
L E F O D P C T 8
9

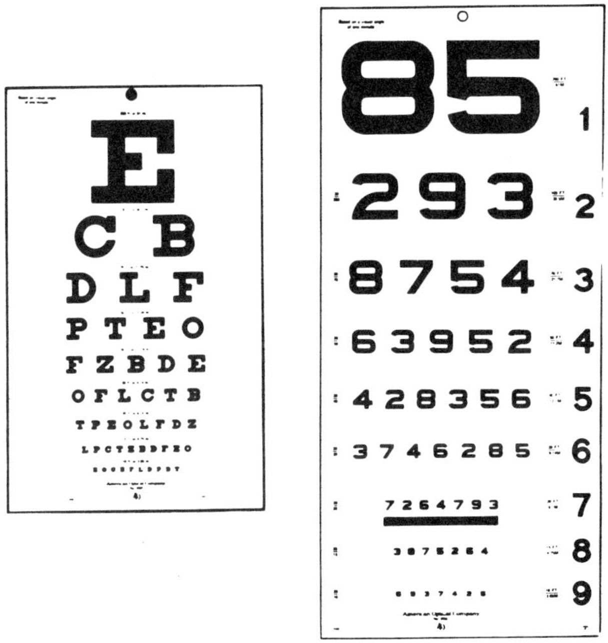

Snellen eye charts. *Better Vision Institute, Inc.*

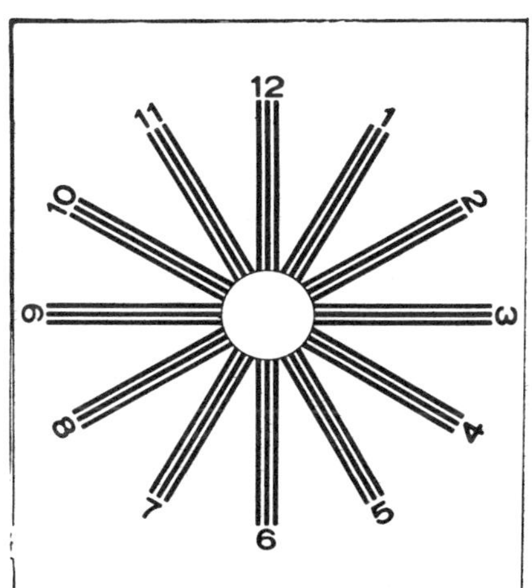

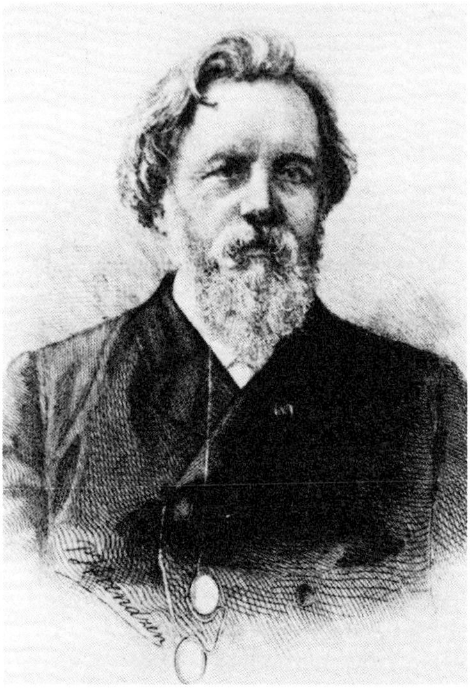

Frans Cornelis Donders

the classic text *On the Anomalies of Accommodation and Refraction of the Eye.* Donders was a precocious, unruly ninth child and his Dutch parents' only boy. He finished lower school and became a tutor at age eleven. Further schooling in his teens taught him Greek, Latin, French, and English. After medical training at Leyden, he became a military surgeon. He was also an accomplished violinist. At twenty-four, the recognition he received from his hard work and his prolific medical writing earned him a teaching job at the University of Utrecht. He added ophthalmology to his subjects in 1847. As his interest grew, he left Holland for the first time to visit the 1851 International Exhibition in London. The fellow ophthalmologists he met there fueled his mounting enthusiasm and led him to establish the Ophthalmic Hospital at Utrecht for treatment and research.

Tall, handsome, genial, Donders was a man whose

time had come. His was the mastermind needed to synthesize fragmented knowledge and bring man's knowledge of ocular refraction from its infancy to a fully developed science. He believed in the use of spectacles, and helped to explode the prevailing theory that wearing them weakened the eyes. "Spectacles are among the most indispensable instruments for man." Everyone who wears well-fitted glasses today is indebted to Frans Donders.

Today you may have your eyes examined by an ophthalmologist, a physician who specializes in eye care and surgery, or by an optometrist, also a licensed eye specialist. Both are qualified to diagnose eye defects and prescribe corrective lenses.

After asking how much close work you do and under what lighting conditions, the specialist will ask you to read the Snellen chart, or he will flash its letters on a

The eye examination. *Better Vision Institute, Inc.*

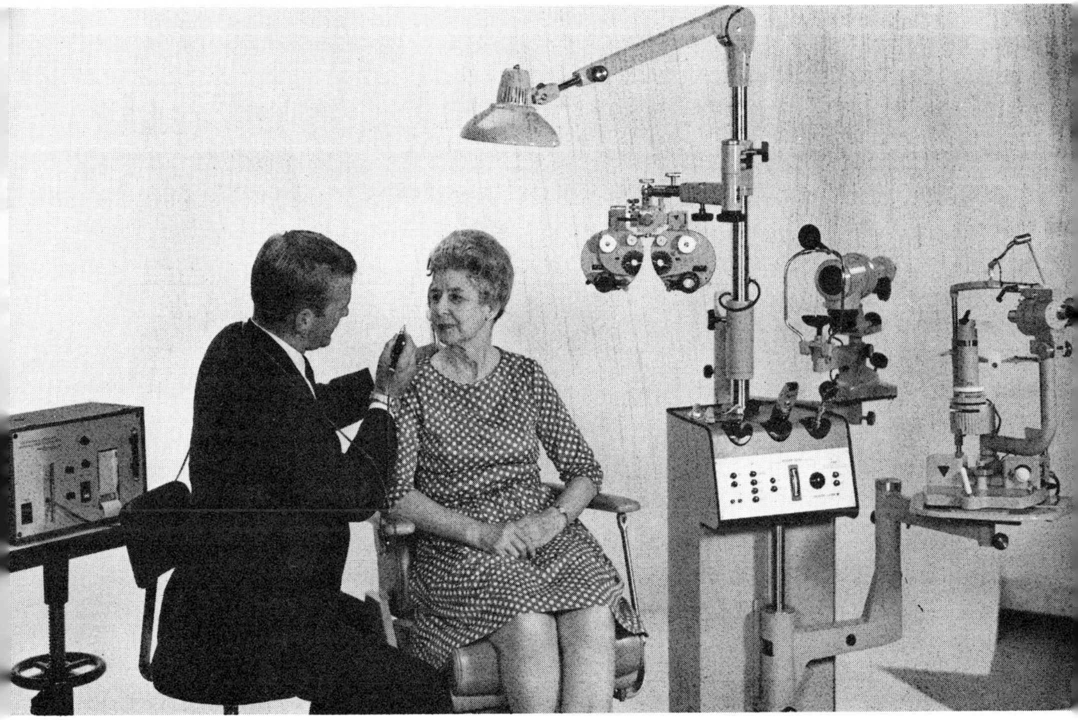

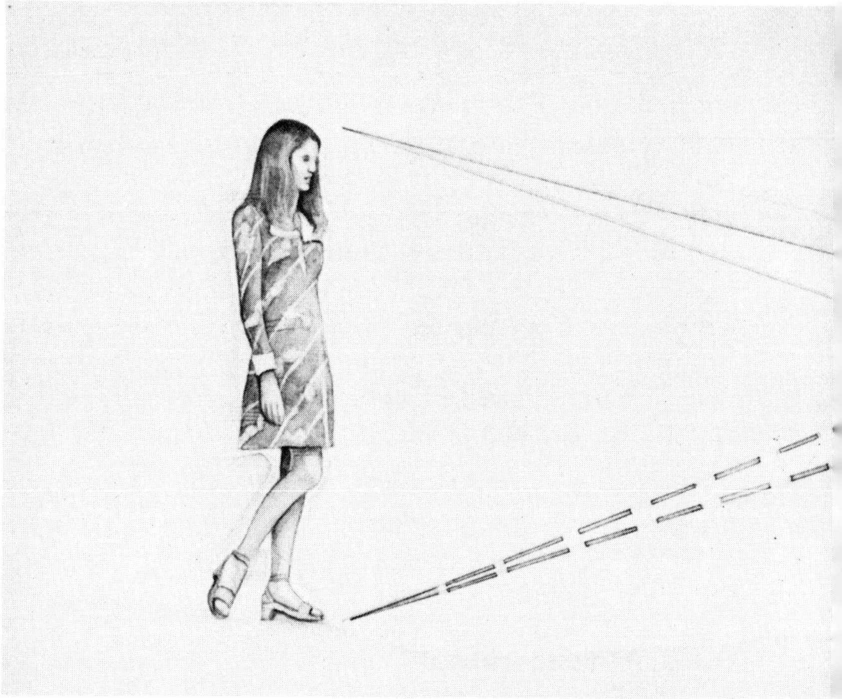

screen. He will test each eye separately for its refractive ability.

One step in the examination will require an ophthalmoscope, a hand instrument invented in 1850 by Hermann von Helmholtz. The ophthalmoscope contains a tiny light bulb, various lenses, and a reflecting prism. By using a sharply focused lens, the examiner can actually see past the reflecting prism into the eye and back to the retina. He can see the arteries and veins along the optic nerve and may detect hardening of the arteries or diabetes as well as certain eye diseases. He can also see a yellow spot at the thickest part of the retina, with a center about 0.5 mm. in diameter. This spot, which is called the fovea, has no blood vessels but holds thousands of cone cells and is the eye's area of most acute vision.

The examiner checks each eye separately. He may use other instruments, such as a retinoscope to measure your near- or farsightedness, or one that determines whether

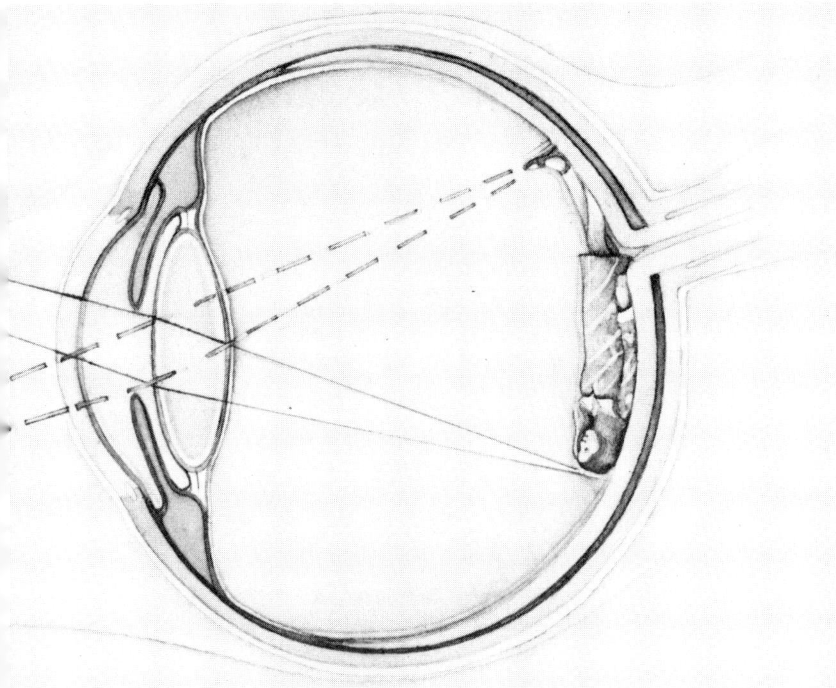

The eye works like a camera

your eyes function in unison. Various charts help him to detect astigmatism and defective color vision.

The final step in the examination is the trial-and-error test to see which lens prescription is best suited for your vision defect, if any. If myopia is your problem, the examiner will prescribe the required concave lens, thicker at the edges than in the center to diverge light rays. For hyperopia, he will prescribe a convex lens, thicker in the center to converge the rays. If he is an optometrist, he can fill his own prescription at your request. Ophthalmologists prescribe, but usually the glasses are supplied by an optometrist or an optician, a dealer in optical supplies.

How does the specialist define the corrective lenses for your eyes? For over two hundred years lenses were marked according to focal length measured in fractions of an inch. Then, in 1872, Monoyer of France introduced what is called the dioptric system. In this code, which specialists adopted early in this century, a prescription will refer to OD (*oculus dexter,* which is Latin for "right eye"); OS (*oculus sinister,* or Latin for "left eye"); OU (*oculus uterque,* or Latin for "both eyes"). The prescription will have a number, followed by *D* for diopter, which is a unit of measurement of lens power. Increasing the power in a convex lens shortens the focus. Increasing the power in a concave lens lengthens the focus. The (+) symbol indicates a convex lens. The (−) symbol means the lens is concave. Additional technical symbols and numbers recommend lens curvature and other requirements.

No examination is complete without a test for glaucoma, a disease caused by a build-up of intraocular pressure that can destroy the optic nerve and the retina. Glaucoma is caused by a failure in the eye's normal drainage system, which allows the aqueous humor to accumulate and reduces the blood supply to retinal nerve cells and the optic nerve. Blindness is the ultimate result. Fortunately, 90 percent of glaucoma patients can be helped by early diagnosis and daily use of eye drops to keep the disease under control.

The test for glaucoma is painless, whether it is done with a hand tonometer to measure the pressure needed to dent the eyeball, or with the more elaborate applanation tonometer, into which the patient looks at one end while the examiner peers through a microscope at the other end to measure the force, sometimes from a puff of air, necessary to flatten a section of the cornea. The examiner checks also for loss of peripheral vision, another symptom of glaucoma. Since the disease is often genetic, persons who have a family history of glaucoma should have this test regularly.

In his book *The Miracle of Vision,* Arthur Freese describes a pliable plastic wafer, Ocusert, which, when slipped under the eyelid, dispenses a continuous supply of pilocarpine, the common drug for glaucoma patients. It needs to be replaced only once a week. The wafer may be uncomfortable for some, but those who can tolerate it will enjoy freedom from the normal every-four-hour routine and avoid the vision blurring caused by drops.

In addition to having regular eye examinations, there are some other sight safeguards. Eyestrain can often be avoided by following the advice of the experts. They warn against these harmful practices:

1. Reading on a moving vehicle. The constant need to refocus puts a strain on the eyes. (An airplane might be an exception.)
2. Reading and writing on a flat-top desk or table instead of on a tilted surface. The tilt provides a direct sight line and saves the eyes from adjusting to the angle distortion.
3. Holding the reading material too close to the eyes. One expert recommends using the Harmon Distance, the minimum distance at which close work should be done. Determine this by measuring from the middle knuckle of your fingers along your arm to the center of your elbow.
4. Watching televison at a distance of less than six feet or in a totally dark room. There should be enough light in the room to neutralize the screen's glare.

What are the most desirable lighting arrangements for reading and writing? Ceiling illumination is ideal, but it may be supplemented by a lamp that shines over the left shoulder for a right-handed individual, or over the right shoulder for the left-handed. Illumination that is limited to a bright, sharply focused lamp can create glare.

Avoid facing a highly colored wall while you are working. A gray or warm white wall is preferable. If a window is your light source, sit so that the window is at your side. A window in front of you will create glare, and one directly behind will cause your shadow to fall on your work. Even then, the glare from bright sunlight may be uncomfortable. If so, it's better to draw the blinds and use only artificial light.

Today eye examinations are a routine part of school health programs. Most adults see an eye specialist regularly. After all, the National Eye Institute ranks visual impairment third in America's chronic diseases, after heart disease and arthritis. Because they are so prevalent, we accept vision defects and corrective eyeglasses as a matter of fact. But what was the reaction when vision aids were first recommended to men and women who needed help?

At first, spectacles were considered by the pious to be a violation of God's natural laws. This view explains the epitaph on Salvino d'Armato's tombstone. But by the sixteenth century they were being sold in the streets, where the buyers selected them by trial and error. Gutenberg's introduction of movable type in the fifteenth century had inspired the masses to literacy and spectacle makers' guilds mushroomed in Frankfurt, Strasbourg, Nurnberg, and elsewhere. Also, physicians were now finally recommending spectacles as a last resort.

Not, however, Dr. Georg Bartisch of Dresden. In 1583 he wrote: "It is much better and more useful that one leaves spectacles alone. For naturally a person sees and recognizes something better when he has nothing in front of his eyes than when he has something there. It is much better that one should preserve his two eyes than that he should have four." Obviously, his patients didn't have a chance.

Although most personal and religious prejudice against spectacles slowly disappeared, a few distinguished critics remained as late as the 1800's. Charles Dickens wrote of spectacles as "something vicious." Goethe, who was extremely nearsighted and sometimes resorted to a lorgnette, expressed his disapproval. "I just cannot help it—but as soon as a man with spectacles enters my room, I feel upset and can hardly overcome my aversion to him. I feel that I am being examined too carefully. I think it is unjust, almost tactless."

John Bunyan rhymed his reluctant acceptance of spectacles:

Spectacles are for sight and not for shew;
Necessity doth spectacles commend,
Was't not for need, there is but very few
That would for wearing spectacles contend.

Schopenhauer refused to wear glasses. So did Jonathan Swift, who confessed that he needed them. He wrote to a friend, "I make nothing of mistaking untoward for Howard; wellpull for Walpole; Knights of share for Knights of shire; monster for minister; in writing speaker I put n for p; and a hundred such blunders which cannot be helped."

But images of spectacles were stamped on coins as early as the sixteenth century—an indication of their respected status. A Danish gold ducat so stamped bears the inscription, "Behold the Wonders of God." A 1589 Brunswick thaler shows the likeness of an old man carrying a torch, an hourglass, a skull, and a pair of spectacles. The translated inscription reads: "Of what avail is lens and light, to him who lacks in mind and might?" A sobering thought.

In 1629, Charles I conferred a royal charter on "Robert Alt on behalf of himselfe and other poore spectacle-makers in and about the Cittie of London," and the Worshipful Company of Spectacle Makers was born. It had strict apprenticeship regulations, and since fines were imposed for "illegally" made spectacles, the Worshipful Company constituted a monopoly. Inferior glasses were publicly smashed upon a large stone opposite the Cannon Street Station, London.

Worshipful Company wardens searched diligently for violations.

> Nicholas Sheild upon search by the Mr. [Master] and Wardens of this Company at his house in ffenchurch streete having found there and he at worke on them eighteene paire of Spectacles being looking glasse wrought onely on the one side and not on the other side for which according to the ordinances he is fined 20s for every paire which is demanded of him here in Court the which he refuseth to pay.

Ultimately, his fine was reduced slightly, and he paid it.

The Worshipful Company took Saint Jerome as their patron saint, an appropriate selection, since Jerome had been painted by Domenico Ghirlandajo (1449–1494) at a desk from which a pair of eyeglasses dangled.

4

Vision Training

Vision training is a phase of eye care that is growing in importance. As a supplement, or, in some cases, a substitute for other vision corrections, it tackles tough problems. To be successful, it requires patience, consistency, and, often, months of cooperation between specialist and patient. Vision training can be helpful to a patient of any age, but is crucial for the vision-impaired child. After all, his visual acuity will govern his ability to read and to adjust to the challenges of school.

A child acquires an immense amount of knowledge even before he enters school. At first, everything a baby grasps goes to its mouth. The tactile and taste senses are at work. The infant learns distance by reaching, sitting, crawling, kicking. Trial and error teach him how near or how far off an object is, whether it is soft or hard, hot or cold. All of this "learning" is recorded in the brain. As one expert put it, the brain is a sophisticated computer. If the wrong information is fed into it at some stage in a child's development (through a vision defect) its answers will be unreliable. Many times this fault can be corrected through therapy.

In vision training, the preschool child is tested for depth perception and color vision along with other visual qualities. Depth perception (stereopsis) is measured by an instrument called a stereopter, and a perception deficiency can often be reduced or corrected by training. Inadequate color vision may require corrective lenses. A color-blind child's path in school will be much smoother if this deficiency is identified early.

For infants or others incapable of participating in eye examinations—the mentally retarded or cerebral palsy victims, for instance—visual-evoked response (VER) provides information about a patient's ocular system from visually evoked brain wave patterns.

Ocular focusing involves coordination of signals from the brain to the eye muscles. When focusing is imperfect or causes strain for any reason, the learning reader will have two strikes against him. Reading proceeds from the reception of an image to recognition or identification and, finally, to comprehension, and the completion of these steps depends on how well the brain is programmed. If a child hasn't learned to integrate touch and vision, or hasn't grasped the concept of directionality, the programming is faulty. Specialists maintain that it can be corrected. Therapy, then, becomes a relearning process. All sorts of

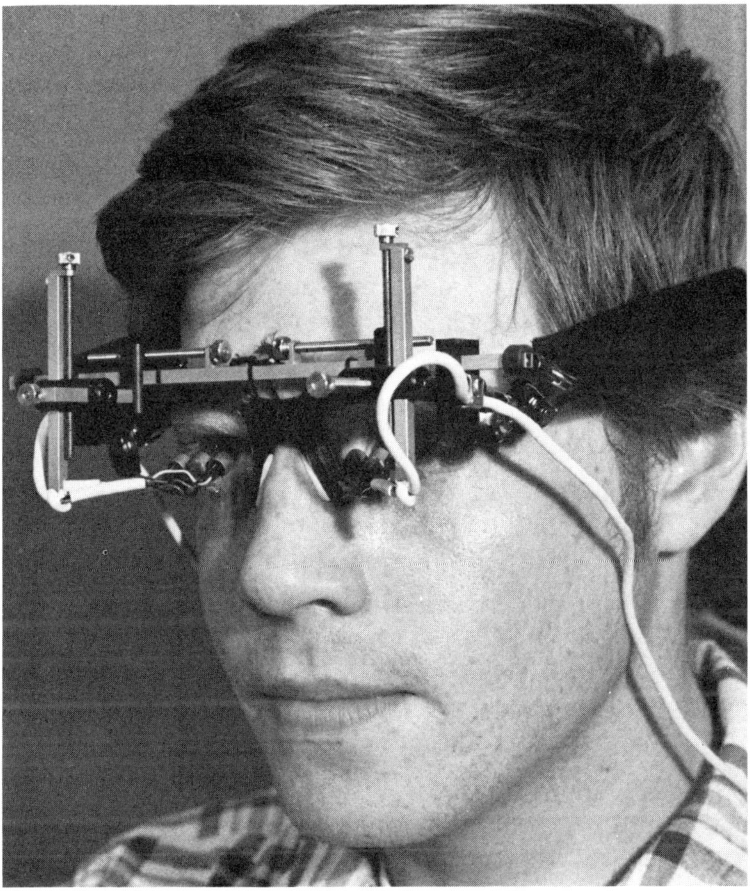

Biofeedback instrument in use at New York State College of Optometry
Stanley G. Goldrich, O.D., Ph.D.

"tools" are used in this process—a variety of lenses, prisms, exercises.

In treating the prevalent defect, strabismus (see Chapter 2), which hampers both children and adults, biofeedback has produced encouraging results. In their book, *Biofeedback*, Karlins and Andrews explain the technique:

> Biofeedback training is the procedure that allows us to tune into our bodily functions and, eventually, to control them. . . . A subject is given this feedback by hooking up with equipment that can amplify one or a number of his body signals and translate them into readily observable signals: a flashing light, the movement of a needle, a steady tone. [Body waves, they say, can then be controlled at will.] Nobody knows why this happens; it just does.

After the initial biofeedback therapy, a strabismus patient learns to sense when he has achieved the desired functioning of the "lazy eye" without a signal. For those who need further help, a portable device may soon be available.

In their book *Out of Sight Into Vision*, Cohen and Shapiro describe visual integrity. Their observations indicate that some individuals are "auditory types" in whom vision and audition can be synthesized in the learning-training process. Others are "tactual types," who rely heavily on the sense of touch. The remainder are the highly visual, whose training can begin on a higher plane, such as judging size, space, form. The highest level is problem solving through visualization, that is, estimating how many steps it would take to cross a room, a street, and so forth.

Vision training is a hopeful approach to correction for many who suffer from crippling sight defects. As the history of this therapy grows, its benefits can be assessed more accurately. The results so far have encouraged specialists and patients alike.

5

Spectacle Lenses, Then and Now

The Babylonian ruler Hammurabi, in his famous Code, granted his subjects permission to use "aids to vision for infirm eyes." We can only speculate as to what these aids were, but we know that the first vision defects were corrected by convex quartz or beryl lenses. In medieval times, journeymen sold them on the streets according to age and sex (women were thought to have weaker vision).

By the seventeenth century tinted lenses were much in favor. Samuel Pepys, diarist and secretary to the admiralty, found his eyesight failing. "I did this evening buy me a pair of green spectacles to see whether they will help my eyes or no. Then to the office and did business till my eyes began to be bad." Unfortunately, Pepys failed to get the desired help and eventually had to abandon his journal.

From the time glass was discovered —probably when drops of pottery glaze accidentally spilled in a baking oven and produced a nontransparent glass—to the transparent blown glass that became the basis for a flourishing industry in Italy by the 1500's, and into the twentieth century, a chain of improvements has led to the present highly refined optical lenses, free of imperfections. One of these improvements occurred in 1805, when cabinetmaker P. L. Guinand, a self-taught optician, tried using a fire-clay stirrer in the manufacture of glass. The long wooden pole previously used had caused ingredients to mix unevenly, forming streaks, but the new stirrer helped produce a much clearer glass.

The ingredients of optical glass (crown glass)—lime, sand, sodium oxide, dry chemicals—have not changed

Pot used for making optical glass *Better Vision Institute, Inc.*

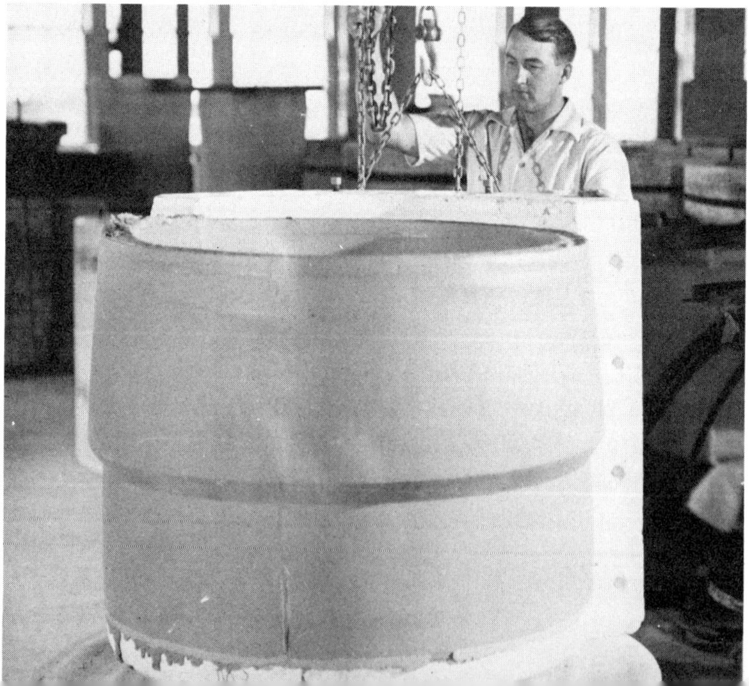

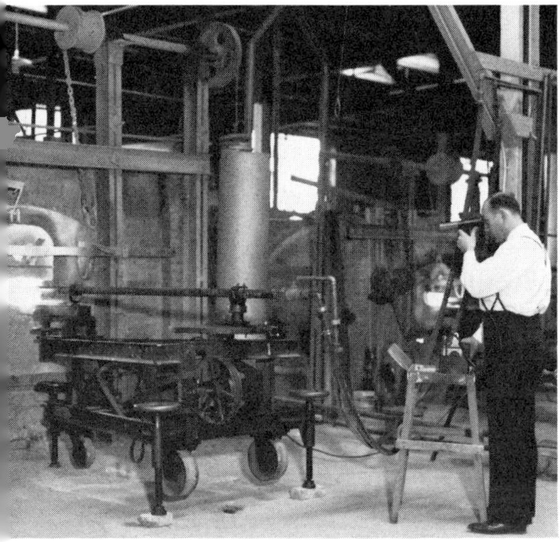

Taking a temperature reading of optical glass in a furnace
Bausch & Lomb Optical Company

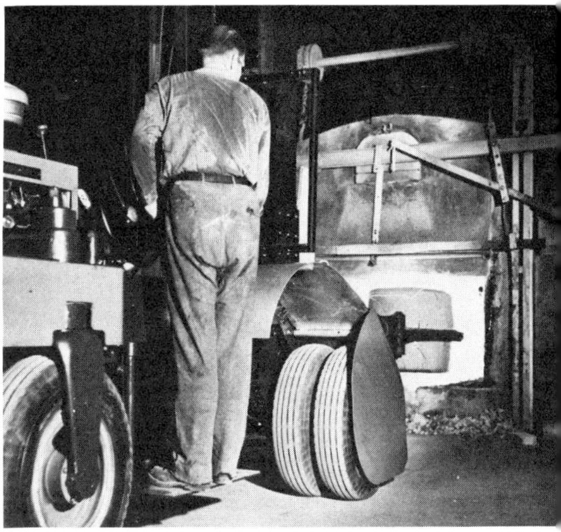

Mechanized equipment moves pot of molten glass from a furnace
Bausch & Lomb Optical Company

much since Guinand's time, and the fire-clay stirrer at the end of a water-cooled tube is still part of what is now an automatic continuous-flow process carried on in platinum-lined tanks. Platinum is used because it does not disintegrate and pollute the melted glass.

Many connecting furnaces are necessary in the continuous-flow process. In the final stage, after periodic checking to eliminate imperfect glass, small amounts are separated out and pressed into rough lens blanks of different curvatures. These blanks go to a last furnace, after which they are slowly cooled in a process called "annealing," and polished. They must be absolutely free of flaws and be of a specific weight before they are shipped to the dispensing laboratories, which stock a variety of uncut lenses.

The laboratories adapt the lenses to individual prescriptions received from optometrists and opticians, a complicated and crucial step. Before the lenses are framed, the pupillary distance (PD) measurement is checked on a lensometer. This procedure establishes that the prescribed

White-hot liquid glass being poured into a rolling table before molding into lenses. *Bausch & Lomb Optical Company*

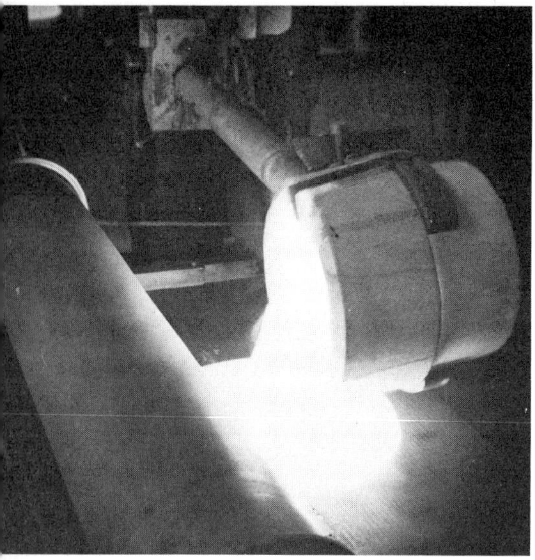

The automatic cylinder surfacer *Better Vision Institute, Inc.*

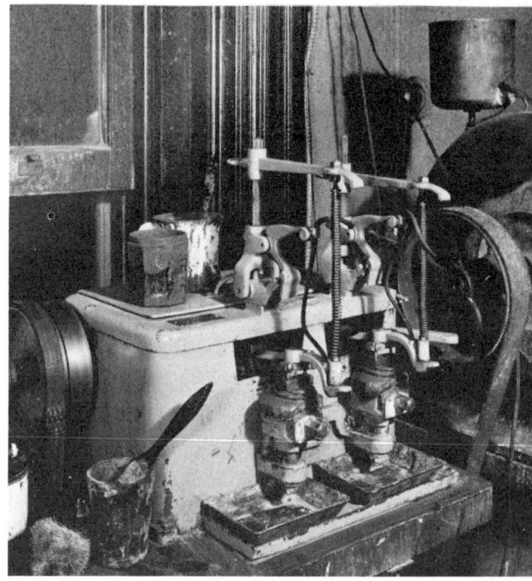

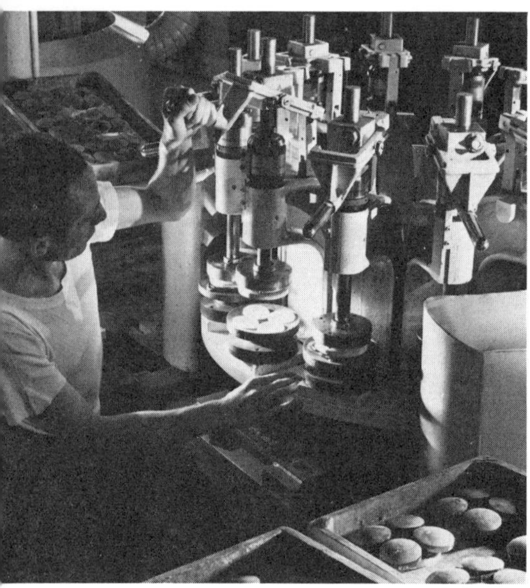

Lens polishing *Better Vision Institute, Inc.*

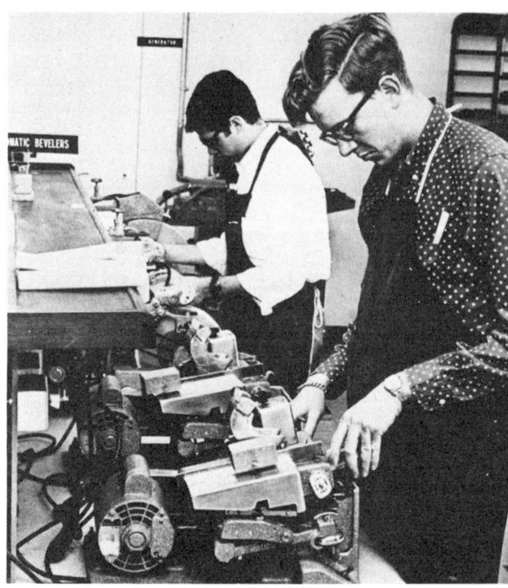

Cutting lenses to size on automatic bevelers *Better Vision Institute, Inc.*

optical centers of the lenses are correct for the wearer. Then, if the lenses conform with government regulations in thickness and shatter-resistance, they are polished and framed.

Optical glass manufacture is highly specialized. Different combinations of ingredients in precise amounts produce special kinds of glass. Some block out ultraviolet rays, others absorb them. Small amounts of optical glass-for tinted lenses, say—are made in fire-clay pots (crucibles), as in the original manufacturing method. Tinted lenses can also be the result of a process called "vacuum deposit" coating, in which they are given a thin covering of a metallic salt.

Before World War I, top-quality optical glass was made only in Europe. But the war forced the American manufacturers to improve their techniques in order to supply large quantities of this type of glass for range finders, submarine periscopes, and other military equipment. Today the United States ranks high in the manufacture of optical glass.

Rough-ground blanks are blocked for another grinding and polishing
Better Vision Institute, Inc.

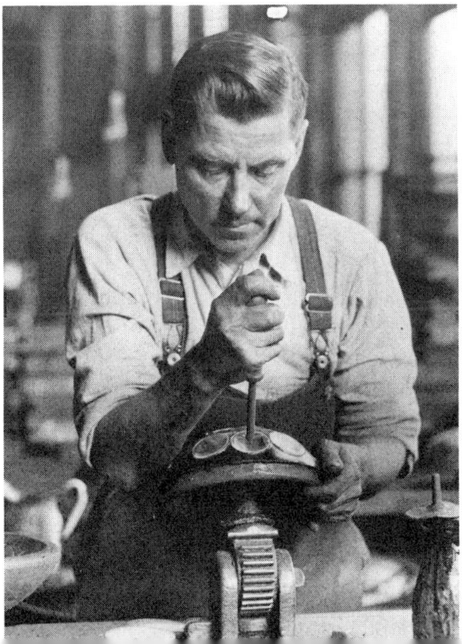

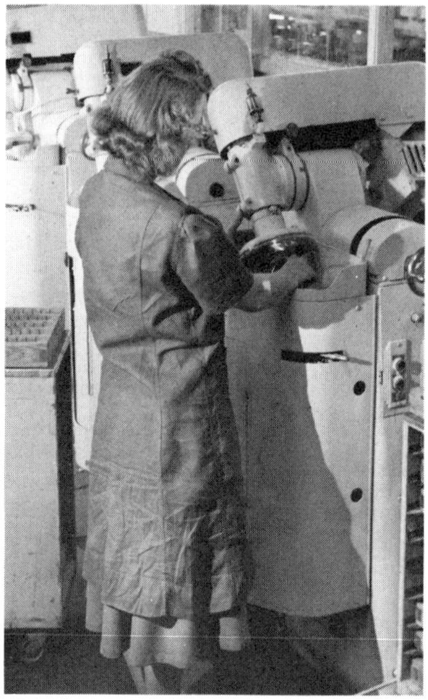

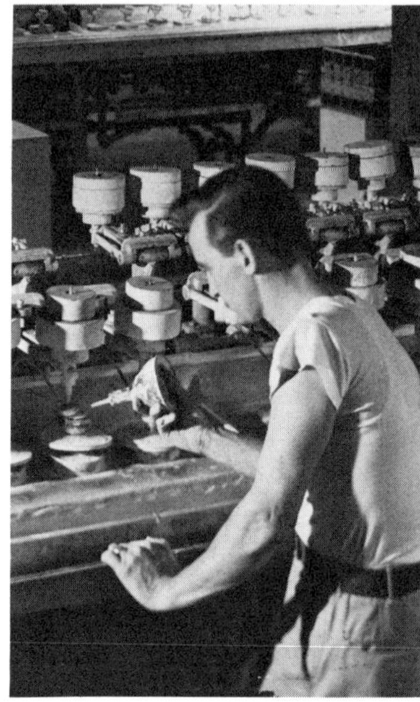

Lens forms are further refined by diamond grinding and polishing
Better Vision Institute, Inc.

Lenses get a final polishing before framing
Better Vision Institute, Inc.

A lens drill
Better Vision Institute, Inc.

The precision spectrometer, used to determine refractive indices of optical glass
Bausch & Lomb Optical Company

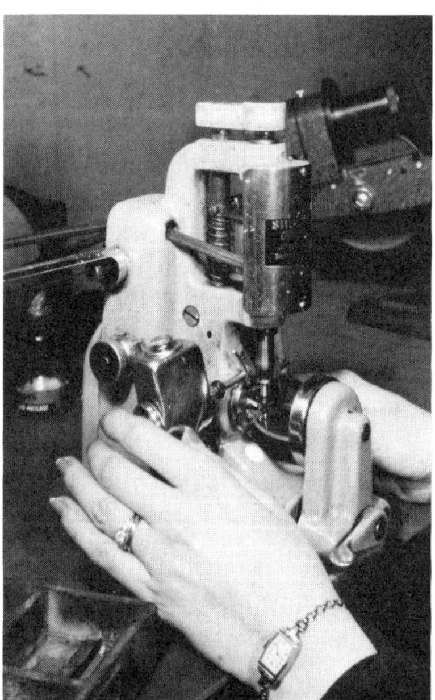

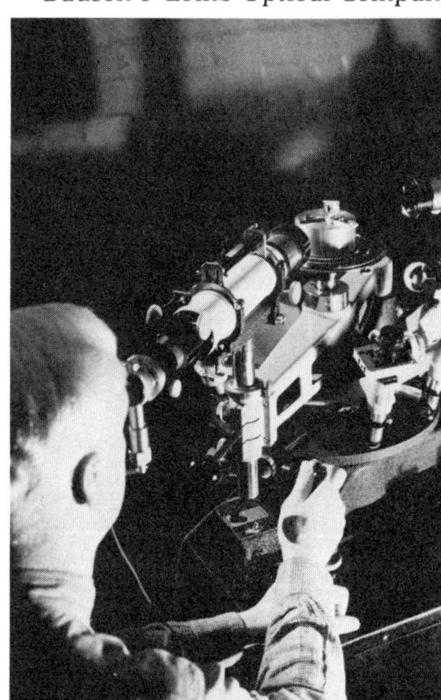

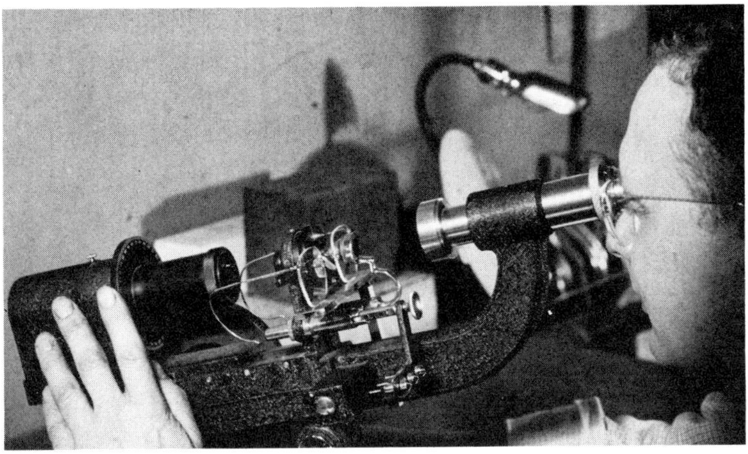

A lensometer measures strength of finished lens and compares it with the original prescription *Better Vision Institute, Inc.*

The earliest reference to a lens measurement was probably that of Jesuit Franciscus Maurolycus (1494–1575), who wrote that "master spectacle makers used to stamp small numbers on spectacles which indicated the age at which they should be worn." These numbers were stamped on the frame. Later, in 1623, a Spanish priest, Daca de Valdes of Seville, originated focal-length measurement. He also wrote a text on optics, benefiting from

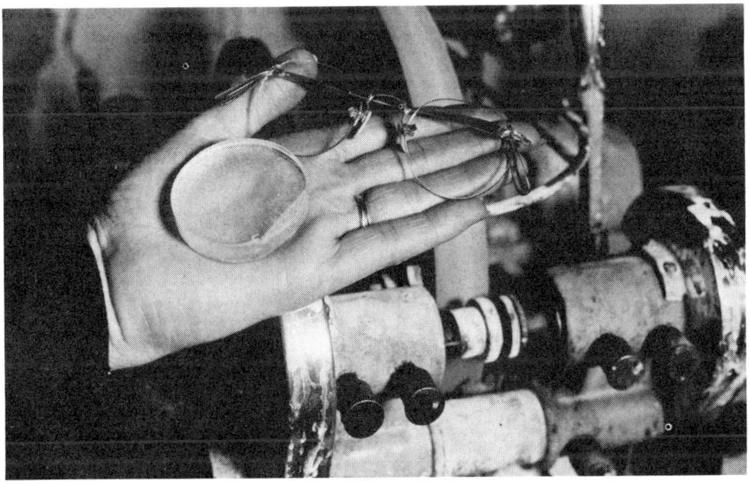

A blank, fresh from the glassmaker, and a finished pair of eyeglasses *Better Vision Institute, Inc.*

the political cooperation then existing between Spain and Holland, where optical glassmaking was far advanced.

Lens measurements fascinated Benjamin Franklin. He wrote to his sister from France in the late eighteenth century:

> I send you a Pair of every size of Glasses from 1 to 13. To suit your self, take a Pair at a time, and hold one of the Glasses first against one Eye, and then against the other, looking on some small Print. If the first Pair suits neither Eye, put them up again before you open a second. Thus you will keep them from mixing. . . . When you have suited your self, keep the high numbers for future Use as your Eyes may grow older; and oblige your Friends with the others.

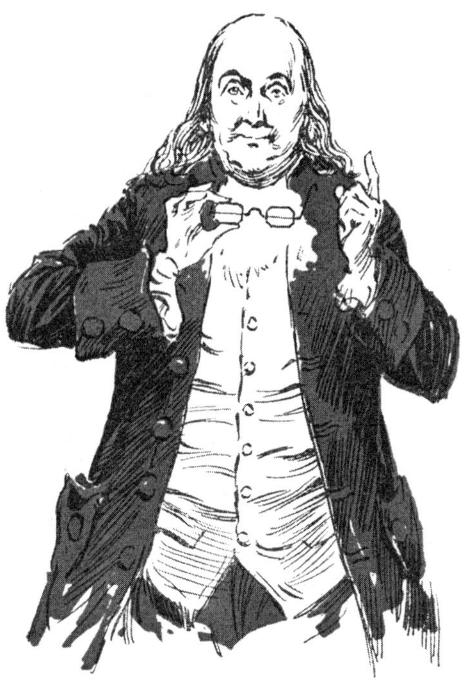

Benjamin Franklin and his bifocals

At about the same time, Franklin wrote to a friend, describing his ingenious improvisation, bifocals. He had combined a half each of a distance and a reading lens in one frame so that "I have only to move my Eyes up or down, as I want, to see distinctly far or near. . . ." But Peter Dollard, Royal Optician by appointment to George III, rejected Franklin's bifocals on the grounds that their use would be extremely limited. Incidentally, if Franklin had not needed a correction for distance, the upper half of his bifocals could have been of plano glass (without optical power) so that he could look up and outward without blurring his vision or removing his glasses. A century later bifocals were fused as we know them. And today lens manufacturers offer a plastic bifocal lens with no visible segment line.

The do-it-yourself fittings of Franklin's time were only a slight improvement over the street vendor's recommendation when spectacles were sold by age. Yet, as recently as 1900, large cities in England had Automatic Eye Testers. They resembled arcade peep-show machines, and operated on the same principle. The tester could peer through a series of lenses and note the number of the lens that best suited him. The "Automatic Sight-Testing and Optical Supply Co." would send the chosen specs on request and receipt of payment.

At first all lenses were flat, causing peripheral vision to be blurred. But thanks to William Hyde Wollaston's research, the curved "periscopic" lens was introduced in 1804. Then an English lens grinder discovered a method of grinding a number of lenses simultaneously, and spectacles were no longer a luxury. Mass production lowered the cost of eyeglasses, making visual help available for almost everyone.

Today all spectacle lenses must be shatter-resistant by federal law. They should be at least 2 mm. thick at the center and heat-hardened. Lighter-weight plastic lenses have proved several times more shatter-resistant than glass. When they were first introduced in 1937, the plastic used was inferior, and production stopped until 1948. By then new developments made plastic a viable material. Hard, thermosetting plastics have been in use since 1960. They are tough, lightweight, almost unbreakable, and fog resistant. The main disadvantages of plastic lenses are a greater susceptibility to scratches and a higher cost.

The first sunglasses in America appeared in the late nineteenth century, and several kinds of tinted lenses were sold after 1872. But, like the tinted spectacles worn in Europe in the seventeenth century, they only reduced glare. The refinement of sunglasses, which today can filter out as much as 90 percent of the light, came much later. Some sunglasses change from light to dark gray as brightness increases. The manufacturers claim that within one minute of exposure to glare these glasses will filter out all but 20 percent of visible light.

Sunglasses protect the eyes, but they are also often worn to create an air of mystery, to relieve tension, or to hide under-eye shadows or other imperfections about which the wearer is sensitive. It is generally agreed by experts, though, that wearing sunglasses indoors can be harmful to the eyes. And, of course, they should never be worn for night driving.

What are the dangers to be aware of when selecting nonprescription sunglasses? Since there are no federal standards except the already mentioned shatter-resistant provision and that of nonflammable frames, the buyer is on his own in the midst of confusion: the inferior and harmful glasses are displayed side by side with the effective, desirable sun-screening glasses.

Specialists warn that plastic sun lenses do not filter out the infrared rays that can burn the retina. Some experts also deplore photochromic sunglasses because they offer too little protection to beach glare and are not effective when worn in a car, because the windshield filters out the ultraviolet rays that activate the lens. The best sunglasses, the experts say, have dark-gray *glass* lenses, which don't distort color. Green or brown glass lenses are second and third choices. Polarized glass lenses, which block out horizontal light vibrations to eliminate glare, are also recommended, but they are expensive.

Here is a test for defective nonprescription sun lenses. Look through each lens at an object such as a window with horizontal and vertical lines. Move the lenses in every direction. If the lines look wavy instead of straight, the lenses are flawed.

6

Frames and Fashions

S*pectacle* wearers fall into three categories. The majority accepts eyeglasses as a necessity. A smaller group self-consciously avoids wearing them in public, and always removes them for photographs. George Washington is reported to have apologized on one occasion, "Gentlemen, you will permit me to put on my spectacles; for, as you see, I have not only grown gray but almost blind in the service of my country." This second group would agree with Dorothy Parker's familiar observation:

Men seldom make passes
At girls who wear glasses.

Those in the third category make the most of the situation. Style-conscious women assemble entire wardrobes of high-fashion specs. Through the years, lens shapes have moved from oval to round to half-size, as fashion dictated. It took several centuries for sidepieces (temples) to evolve, but countless frame styles have followed each other during the past fifty years. Most of them are revivals. As in clothing, long-forgotten styles often return, to be greeted as innovations.

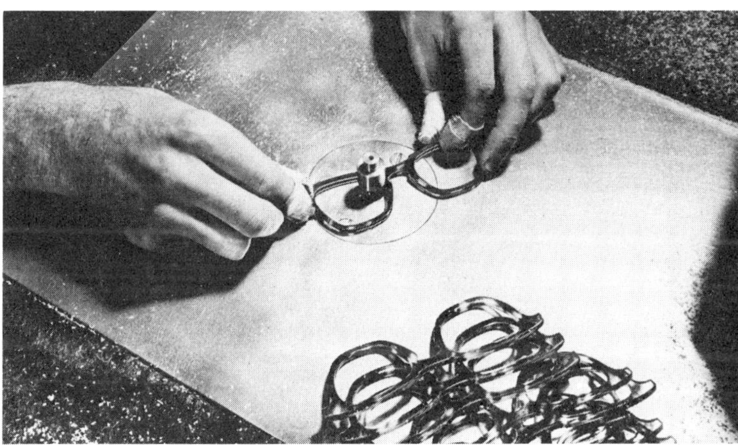

Grooving operation during zyl (plastic) frame manufacture
Better Vision Institute, Inc.

Public-relations writers have tried in the past to establish rules for the most-becoming glasses. According to *Fashion's Glass*, a publication of the Better Vision Institute, angular lenses counteract mooniness in a round face; the symmetry of round or oval lenses counteracts irregularity of feature; straight-sided lenses lessen the prominence of high cheekbones and facial fullness. These writers also recommend specific glasses for different activities: for sports, business, dancing, bridge, motoring, etc. Etiquette authority Emily Post once declared: "The right eyewear at the right time and place—this is the final test of good taste for the discriminating woman."

Today, too, how you look is as important as what you look through. One optician, specializing in "Unusual Frames for Unusual People," offers in his advertisement to photograph a prospective customer wearing "our fashionable frames" so she can see how she looks. Dress designer Diane von Furstenberg and other fashion designers lend their names to high-fashion eyewear. This is not an altogether new idea. In a 1925 radio address on "Glasses and Appearance," John F. Hill reported: "Not long ago I saw illustrated in one of our leading fashion magazines a group of beautiful glasses, which had been created by a great French designer."

Today's heady variety of frames and lens shapes and style-conscious promotions are really an old story. In 1701, when the Spanish king Philip V and his wife, Marie-Louise of Savoy, entered Madrid, her five hundred ladies-in-waiting *all* wore tortoise-shell-framed spectacles. Tortoise shell was a favorite because of its light weight. The tortoise was sacred in China, and such frames were thought to bring good luck.

Experiments in spectacle design were endless. Coats of arms decorated bridge pieces; a pair of Indian specs displayed two facing elephants of carved sandalwood on an arched nosepiece; lenses were concealed in fans, behind which flirtatious eyes sought admirers. Gentlemen had lenses in walking sticks and on watch fobs. The rich demanded ornate frames of gold or other expensive materials and the most sophisticated workmanship.

Rich or poor, everyone had difficulty keeping spectacles in place. In Rabelais' *Gargantua*, Panurge wore spectacles attached to his hat. Sir Thomas More let his glasses ride on the lower part of his nose. Henry VIII's court jester,

Will Somers, had a suit of armor with spectacles riveted to the helmet. El Greco's portrait of Cardinal Niño de Guevara shows him wearing glasses attached to the ears by loops of cord. Glasses could also be tied around the head by leather or ribbon straps. One uncomfortable-sounding seventeenth-century design, the forehead frame, which, of course, was worn around the forehead, had a metal band to which steel frames were riveted.

Temples, introduced in 1728 by Edward Scarlett of London, were a step in the right direction. Sir Joshua Reynolds, the famous portrait painter, had elegant silver wig spectacles with temples that could be extended. These may have been less secure, but they were surely more agreeable than the 1735 model with temples of iron, ending in circular clamps, even though occasionally these clamps were mercifully covered with velvet.

In addition to nose glasses, there were monocles (preferred by Napoleon, who was myopic), lorgnettes (worn by Marie Antoinette), quizzers, and other single glasses. A single glass on a ribbon, called a "young glass," or a "perspective glass," was fashionable for distance viewing in the seventeenth century.

The quizzer has a confused identity. Some have described it as a version of the monocle; others claim it was a mirror through which its owner could follow activities going on behind him while seeming to look straight ahead.

"*La lorgnette bienséante,*" the becoming lorgnette, also called the jealousy lorgnette, was a favorite of Mme. Pompadour. It resembled one half of an opera glass and had an oblique mirror. By looking into the mirror through a hidden hole in the side decoration, the viewer could see hanky panky to the rear or to the side: an excellent way to keep track of one's rivals. It should be understood that the French lorgnette resembled a small telescope. Its counterpart in England, called "a prospect glass," was a precursor of the opera glass.

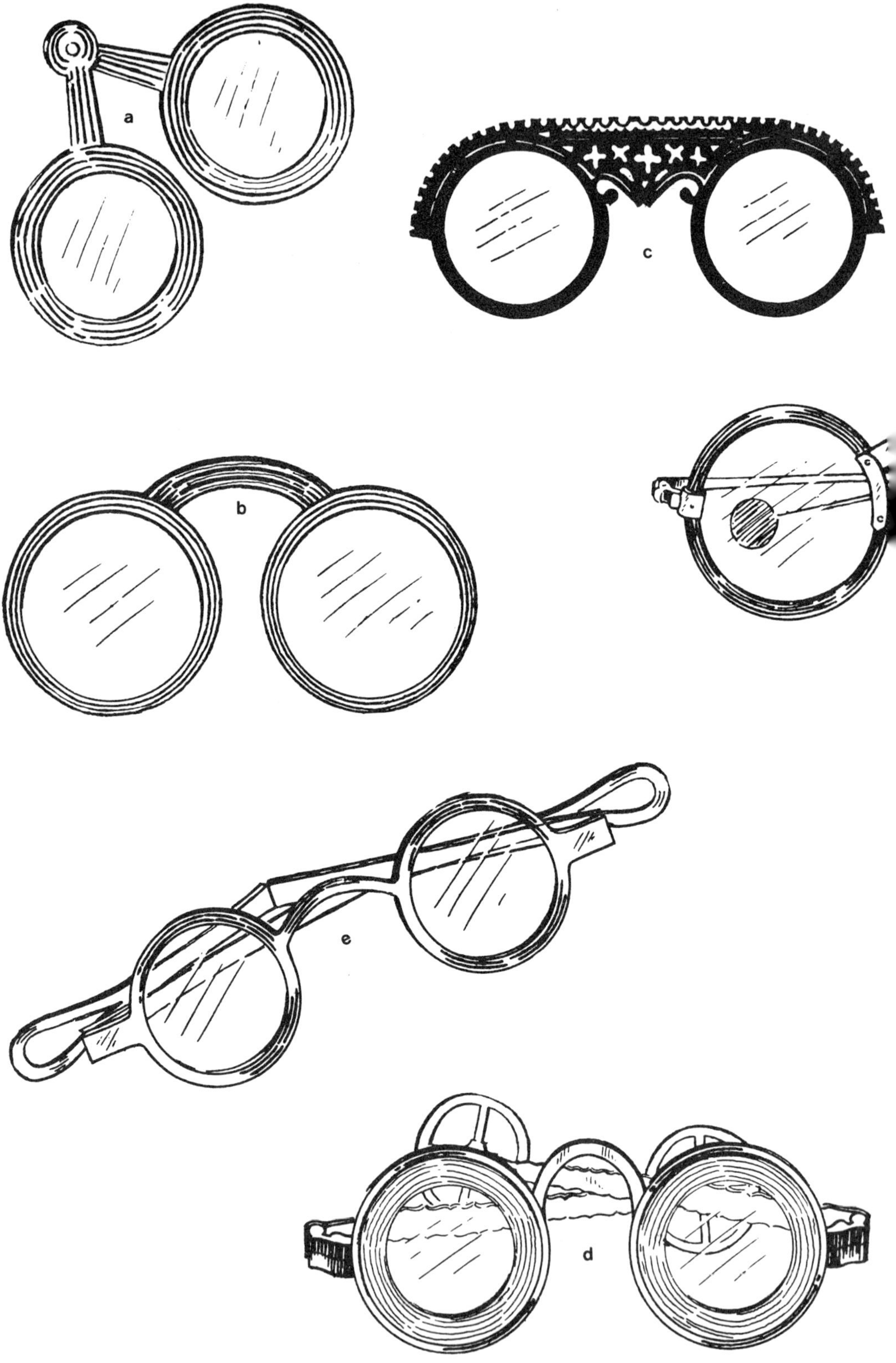
a
c
b
e
d

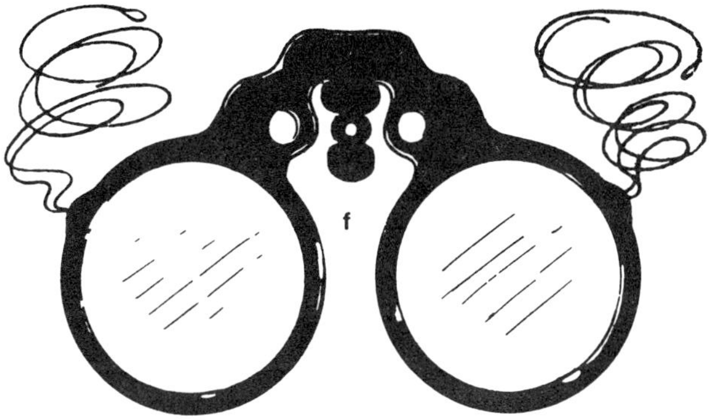

f

g

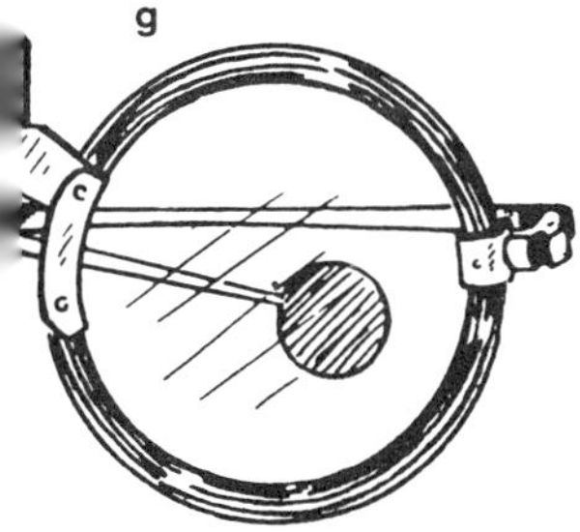

a. Eyeglasses of the 1300's. The frame is of bone and pivots on a rivet. They clamped on the nose.

b. Eyeglasses typical of the 1500's—of horn, with bridge constructed to give it "spring."

c. German eyeglasses of about 1650. Some had holes in the rims, through which cord was strung and looped over the ears.

d. In the early 1700's spectacles were invented with metal sides ending in large loops that clamped against the temples. These are of iron, with inner rims of horn.

e. George Washington wore these spectacles. They have hinged sides ending in loops. A ribbon could be run through the loops to tie the spectacles on.

f. Chinese spectacles. Tortoise-shell rims with cord earpieces and movable carved nosepiece; used in China 250 years ago.

g. Old Chinese spectacles. Rims of horn; sides hinged, with solid round ends for clamping against the head.

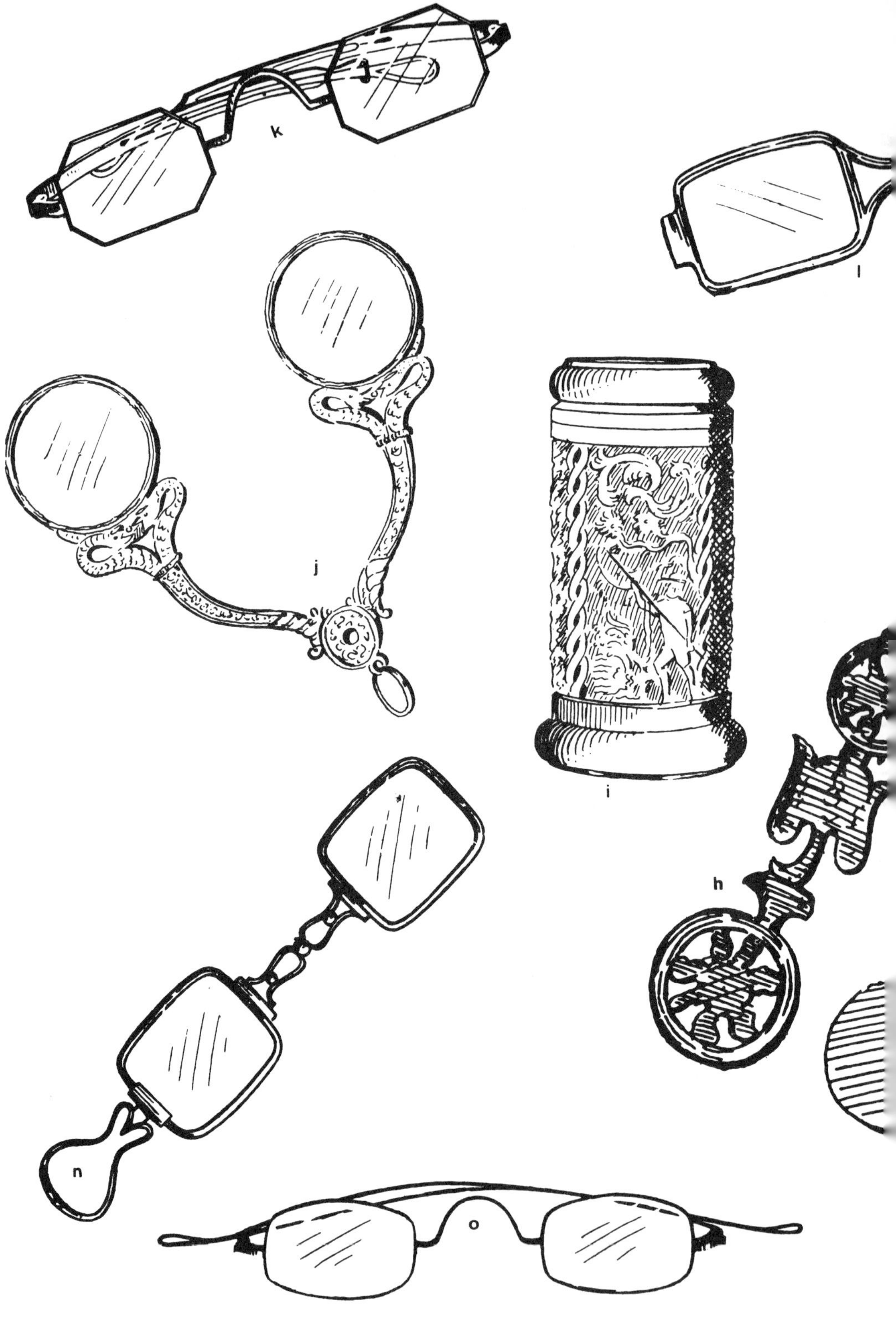
k
l
j
i
h
n
o

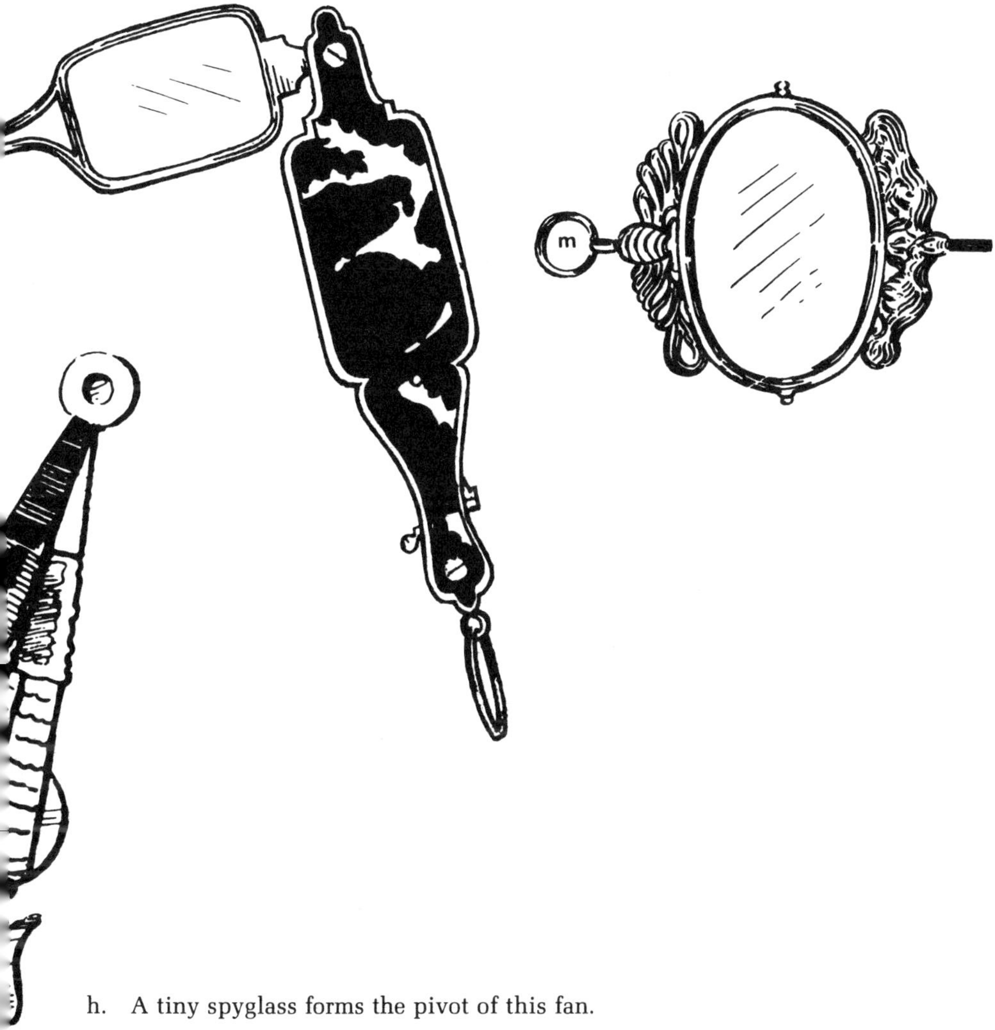

h. A tiny spyglass forms the pivot of this fan.

i. An ivory lorgnette of pre-Revolutionary France. It was in reality a "spyglass," used for distance seeing.

j. This "wishbone" lorgnette has elaborate arms of silver and is of a style popular in France under the Directoire.

k. Spectacles of 1800, with sliding earpieces adjustable in length.

l. Tortoise-shell-and-gold lorgnette with a hinged bridge. About 1830.

m. A "quizzer," or "monocle for the hand," popular in the middle 1800's. This one embodies its owner's watch key.

n. Folding gold lorgnette with pivot bridge. About 1848.

o. Spectacles of 1860, with hair-thin frame of blue steel wire.

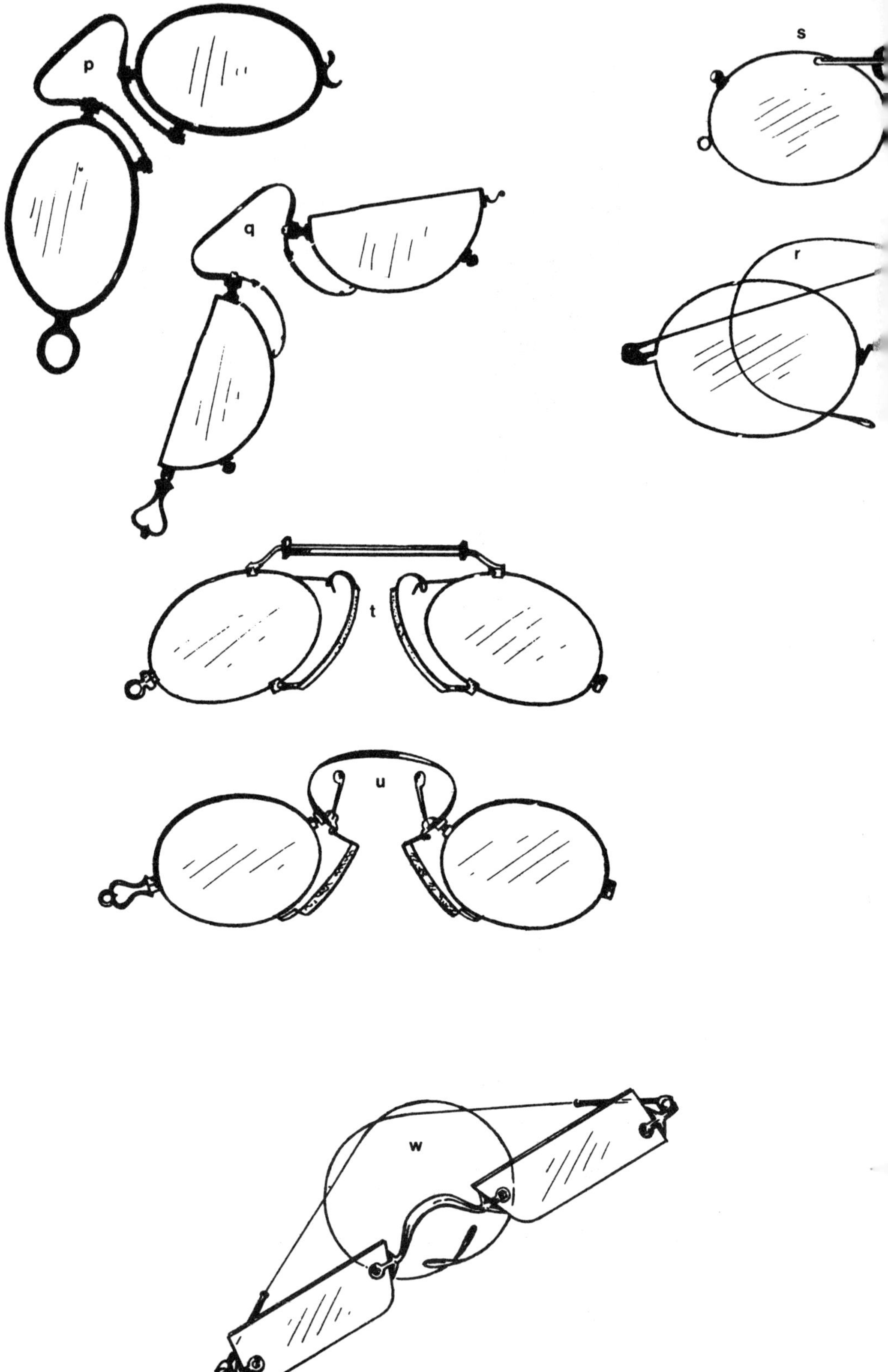
p
q
s
r
t
u
w

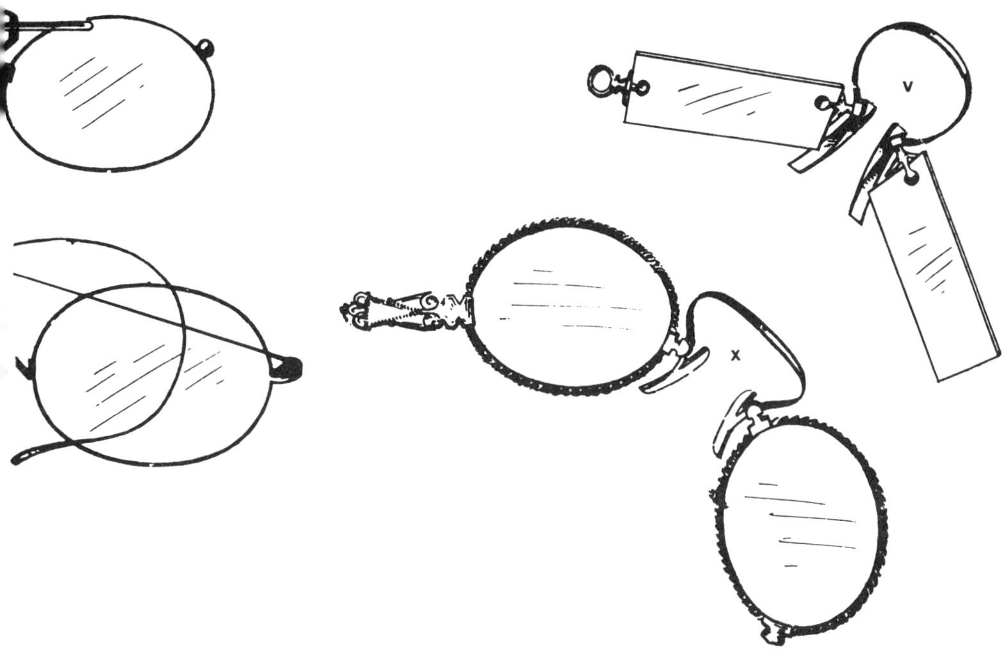

p. Folding oxford of 1875, with rims of thin shell and bridge of flat blue steel.

q. Another style of oxfords of 1875, with flat blue steel nose spring and lenses rimmed with hair-thin blue steel.

r. The first of the "modern" spectacles. Thin wire frames of blue steel; sides that curve behind the ears.

s. Quaint old eyeglasses with fan-shaped, cork-faced nose-guards and reinforced nose-bridge.

t. Old French eyeglasses, pince-nez, rimmed with silver; cork nose-guards and intricate spring bridge.

u. Two little prongs to fit in the eyepits helped hold these old eye-glasses at the proper angle.

v. Old French pince-nez eyeglasses with cork guards and high arched silver bridge.

w. Old French rimless spectacles, with tiny lenses; ribbon bridge and earpieces of silver.

x. An oxford of about 1900, finely wrought in solid gold with gadroon-engraved rims.

Better Vision Institute, Inc.

It was very much the fashion to use a lorgnette in public, but this practice troubled an 1870 writer in a book on decorum:

> The functions of the natural eye and eyeglasses are much abused. . . . Nothing can be more ill bred, and we assert it in the face of assenting fashion, than ogling a stranger in the streets through an eyeglass—with a stony British stare—or surveying an opposite neighbour at the theatre with a lorgnette.

In Colonial America all specs were imported. Some cost as much as two hundred dollars. The *Boston Evening Post* carried an advertisement in 1756 with an illustration of a pair of glasses:

> Just imported in the Scow Two Brothers, Cpt. Marsden, from London and to be sold by Hannah Breitnall at the Sign of the Spectacles, in the Second Street near Black-Horse-Alley. Variety of the finest chrystal spectacles, set in temple, steel, leather, and other frames. Likewise true Venetian green spectacles for weak or watery eyes, of various sorts. Also concave spectacles for short sighted persons, magnifying and reading glasses.

As early as 1893 the president of the ophthalmological section of the British Medical Association was hoping that "we may ultimately reach a position in which a man who goes about with his eyes naked will be so rare that the sight of him will almost raise a blush." No British reserve there.

The Empire Bible and Spectacle Institution of Tiverton offered a "Philanthropist's Parcel" containing "1 dozen good spectacles, ages assorted, 1 dozen cases, 1 dozen Gospel books, and 3 copies of the Gospel in 3 dozen foreign languages, all post paid in wooden cases for 36 penny stamps to any address in the United Kingdom."

Greater changes in eyeglasses have come about in the twentieth century than occurred in the previous six. Plastic made a big difference; bifocals, trifocals, and quadrifocals were perfected; contact lenses became accepted eyewear. Dr. Norburne B. Jenkins, writing in 1900 in the *Optical Journal,* had discouraged any unnecessary use of spectacles. "Glasses are very disfiguring to women and girls," he wrote. But within a decade, a majority of both sexes was enthusiastically trying each new version of specs that appeared.

Spectacles in America had been difficult to keep in place until 1880, when the first ones appeared with curved steel temples that fit snugly over the ears to hold them in place.

Oddly, just when the problem was solved, a new style called "oxfords" was introduced. They had *no* sidepieces, but were held in place by a springy nosebridge. When not in use, these spectacles dangled from a ribbon or cord attached to the wearer's clothing, although some people preferred to store their oxfords on a chain which, reellike, curled into a round button. Teddy Roosevelt wore oxfords, and later, Calvin Coolidge, too. They were also called pince-nez. All of them had nose pads attached to the bridge piece, which was controlled by tiny coil springs that gripped the nose.

In 1950, a reporter, who had worked part time as a lens grinder, advised Senator Robert A. Taft to change from the rimless glasses with metal nosepiece and metal temples, which made him look like a schoolteacher, to shell-rimmed glasses. Taft took his advice, and joked that if he'd done it years before, he might have been elected President.

In *Holiday* magazine, Hugh Foster wrote:

> Dwight D. Eisenhower saw himself through eight years in office on only two changes of glasses. He came in wearing the gold-rimmed Dean-of-Men model he had acquired at Columbia University and went out in a pair of clear plastic Dynamics. President Truman went through three changes, beginning with Missouri Gothic, switching midway

through his first term to the rimless, octagonal Merchant Prince and finally to the modified Clubman.

Out of this history of spectales has come an intriguing by-product—collecting.

The collector of antique eyeglasses leads an interesting life. His hobby may also turn out to be profitable. With expertise, real finds are possible in unexpected places. Optometrist L. D. Bronson, an authority on antique specs, reports the purchase by one of his patients of a "silver-colored lorgnette." She had paid $7.35 for it at an antique show. Dr. Bronson examined it with a compound magnifier and discovered that the "silver" material was actually platinum and that the lorgnette was worth at least $250. But he advises caution if a specimen costs more than $25, because many replicas are now available.

Dr. Bronson gives an interesting example of the appreciation of a pair of spectacles that were priced in the 1912 Sears-Roebuck catalog at $2.60. In 1966, these spectacles were worth $5.50, and antique shops recently offered $50 to $75 for the same ones. A gold lorgnette Bronson paid $15 for in 1960 is now priced above $150.

Old spectacle cases, he says, can be equally valuable. Many are set with pearls and gem stones. An 1880 Spencer catalog listed "Silk Plush Chatelaine cases at $7.50 per dozen." Present prices for these cases range from $15 to $200 *each*.

Who knows what treasure may be discovered at the bottom of an old trunk in a corner of the attic?

7

Contacts

When Leonardo da Vinci, that tireless experimenter, submerged his face in a glass bowl filled with water in 1508, the bowl became the refracting surface for his eye, while the water served as the tears between the glass and the cornea. In principle, Leonardo had devised a kind of contact lens, which was suggested again 300 years later by English astronomer Sir John E. Herschel.

Although the use of contacts has suddenly mushroomed, especially since soft lenses were introduced, the

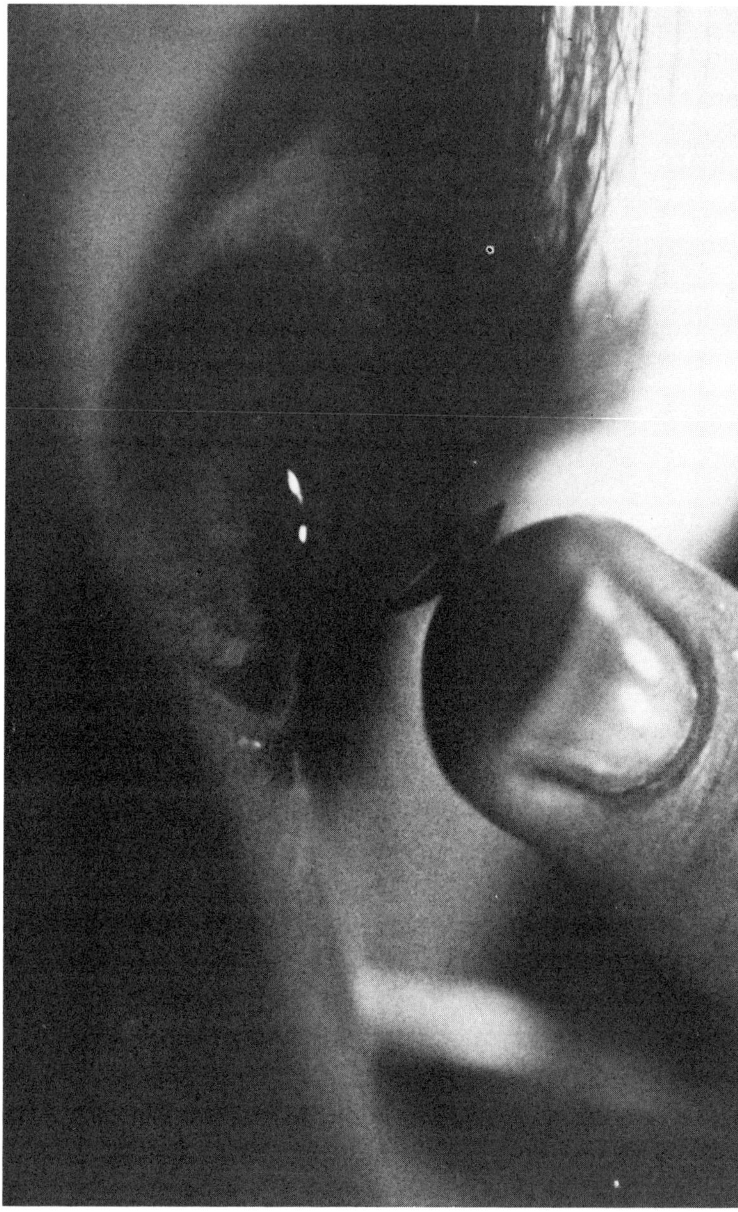

Inserting a contact lens *Better Vision Institute, Inc.*

first ones, of glass, were tried without much success in 1887 by the German physiologist A. E. Fick. In 1938 there was revolutionary development in contacts, when the plastic methyl methacrylate made hard contact lenses widely acceptable. Now many different plastics are used. By 1958, bifocal contact lenses were available, and in 1970 soft, hydrophilic (water-absorbent) plastic lenses added another choice to vision aids.

Contact lenses, worn today by more than five million persons, have none of the inconvenience of traditional eyeglasses. They also provide a wider field of vision, and, for those who suffer from scarred or irregularly shaped corneas, they may be the only answer to sight defects. For others, contacts represent a safe, cosmetic solution to their vision problems. More than half of this country's professional athletes wear soft contacts; 33 percent of them wear hard contact lenses; and 14 percent, mostly baseball players, wear eyeglasses.

The rocketing popularity of contacts brings dangers and warnings for the uninitiated. Beware of the semi-trained advertiser and seller of contact lenses. The secret to satisfaction is precise fitting by a licensed optometrist and, often, repeated visits for adjustment during the breaking-in period. The wearer should have complete information about the care of his lenses. He should know what the time span is for safe and comfortable wearing and what to do if discomfort occurs. Some people should not try to wear them at all. The expert can explain why, if this is true.

The earliest contacts were scleral. They covered the white, opaque portion of the eye (the sclera), and required a special fluid between the lens and the sclera. But in 1950 a smaller corneal lens became popular. Often only one-third inch or less in diameter and one-hundredth of an inch thick, the lens remains in place by capillary attraction to the cornea's tear film. No other fluid is required.

Today, with a choice between hard and soft contacts,

only the wearer, with the advice of a specialist, can decide which to select. Both types must preserve the healthy condition of the cornea, which needs access to oxygen and nutrients from the air and the eye's tears. When the lens is fitted, its curvature, size, thickness, and edge beveling must provide leeway for the outward passage of used tear fluid and its replacement with fresh tears. Some contacts have tiny holes to achieve this exchange.

Many who were unable to wear hard contacts have welcomed the soft lenses. They are usually comfortable and almost never fall out. They prevent dirt from getting to the cornea, and are better for night driving because they reduce glare or sparkle. But soft lenses have disadvantages. They are not yet a good correction for astigmatism, and may provide only variable vision. Since they are absorbent, they must be cleaned of pollutants from the air and from ocular-fluid fats and proteins, in addition to being sterilized daily. They may rip, tear, or discolor, and a prescription cannot be reground. They have a short life span and are more expensive than hard contacts.

Although all contacts can be worn for only limited periods, experiments in long-term wearing are afoot. The extended-wear lens has not been approved by the Food and Drug Administration, which, along with many specialists, deplores the competitive rush to achieve its acceptance. But a hard, cellulose-acetate material, which manufacturers claim to be permeable to oxygen and carbon dioxide, is being tried, and, according to a recent report, one contact-lens technician has worn these gas-permeable lenses since Labor Day, 1973, and has taken them out only a few times to remove dirt particles.

Soft contact lenses provide both therapeutic and cosmetic protection. They can shield the surface of an injured or diseased cornea and can keep medication in place after surgery or in the case of ocular burns. In myopia, a condition resulting from an abnormal curvature of the cornea, or a too-long eyeball, hard contacts are sometimes used in a procedure called orthokeratology, which employs them in successively flatter forms to reshape the cornea. Many specialists have strong reservations about the treatment, which has very little history, and has not yet been sufficiently tested.

Contacts have earned a wide acceptance for use after cataract surgery, which is performed mostly on persons over age sixty. In spite of considerable research, ophthalmologists still don't know what causes cataracts, and cannot treat them effectively. Surgery is the only answer when vision is impaired.

In ancient times, "needling" or "couching" meant loosening the obstruction behind the iris of a cataract patient with a needle. The obstruction then dropped into the back of the eye. Finally, in the eighteenth century, autopsies revealed that the "obstruction" was actually the eye's diseased lens.

Today the diseased lens is removed through a small incision at the edge of the cornea. But when the natural lens has been removed, unfocused light reaches the retina and causes blurring, and post-operative eyeglasses not only magnify greatly but provide little side vision. Contact lenses reduce the magnification markedly and widen the field of vision.

But what about the elderly, the unsteady, the victims of rheumatoid arthritis or Parkinson's disease, who cannot manage contacts? For them, surgeons are implanting plastic lenses at the rate of 7500 a year. During World War II, a British professor of ophthalmology observed that British flyers seemed to tolerate bits of plastic that lodged in their eyes from shattered airplane windows. This inspired the experiments leading to today's implants.

Immediately after the operation to remove a diseased lens, a soft plastic contact lens is attached to the pupil with nylon clips. Dr. Norman S. Jaffe, of the University of Miami

School of Medicine, says that of his 450 recent implants on patients whose average age was 74.3 years, 90 percent achieved 20/40 or better vision. He cautions against implants for younger patients until more studies have been made over a long term. Jaffe warns that anyone considering a lens implant should seek a surgeon with extensive experience in this field.

The use of soft contacts has expanded rapidly. As research continues, a breakthrough will undoubtedly occur and introduce new possibilities for contacts as vision aids. Several families of oxygen-permeable materials are now appearing in lens form. These materials may provide a solution to the problems inherent in fitting to the corneal surface a comfortable, corrective lens that can be worn indefinitely.

8

The Three O's

Ophthalmologists, Optometrists, Opticians

In *the* nineteenth century in America eyeglasses were often fitted by storekeepers. Abraham Lincoln is reported to have stopped at a jewelry store one day on his way to the Bloomington, Illinois, railway station to spend 37½ cents for his first pair of spectacles. On the 1976 anniversary of Lincoln's birth, the items that were found in his pockets when he was assassinated, and which had been preserved in a sealed container, were revealed for the first time. They included two pairs of spectacles.

The world's first optometry law was passed in Minnesota in 1901. It was designed to protect the public from exploitation by "travelling opticians" and "spectacle peddlers." The Minnesota law provided for a board appointed by the governor, an examination fee of ten dollars, a five-dollar fee for the issuance of a certificate to practice optometry, and an annual license fee.

Widespread optometry legislation had been delayed, because ophthalmologists, who had M.D. degrees, were reluctant to recognize the role of optometrists. Dr. Thomas Hall Shastid, an ophthalmologist, reported near the turn of the century:

Selecting a pair of spectacles at the general store in the 1800's

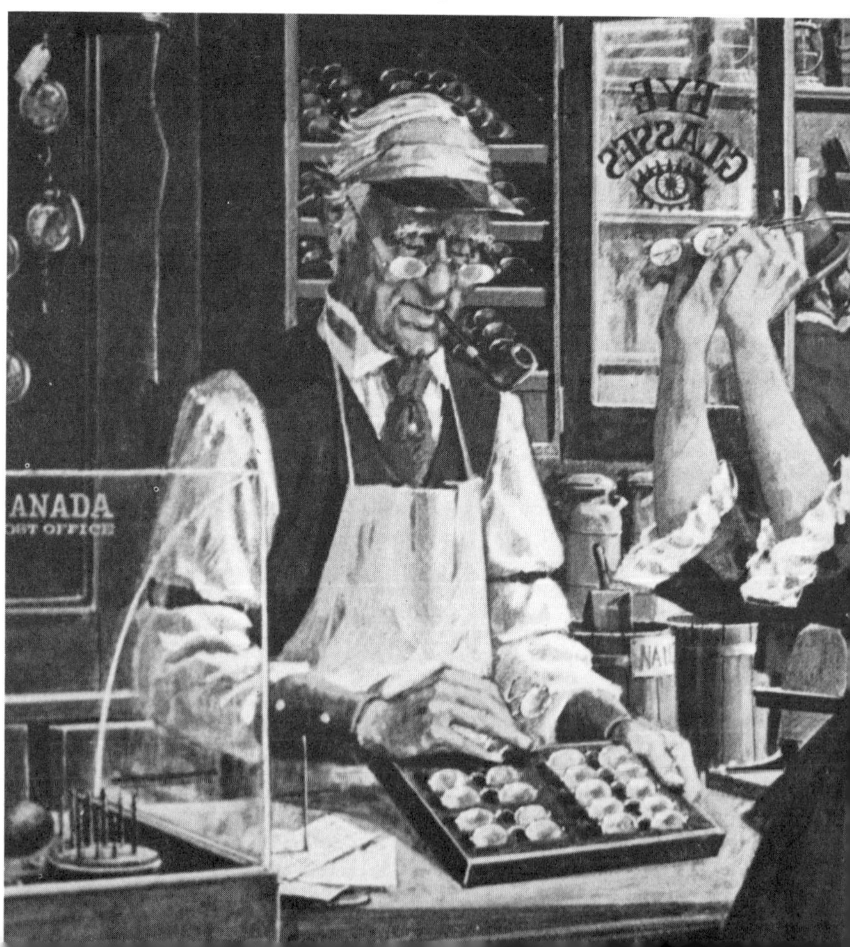

> There were certain traveling "spec-peddlers" who went from house to house fitting glasses, and unskillful though they were, relieving many of the simpler cases of eyestrain, headache, sick stomach and nervous disorders. Such men . . . excited extreme contempt and bitterness on the part of the "regular" profession, feelings which grew the more the "spec-peddler" beat the scientific M.D.'s at the treatment of eyestrain and its numerous results. . . . Hardly anything that now I can recall served so much to weaken the standing and influence of physicians in any community than this absurd, ridiculous, hard-headed, stubborn, absolutely unyielding opposition to the fitting of glasses for anything whatever except simply and solely the difficulty known as "old sight."

Hilco, a Division of the Hilsinger Corporation

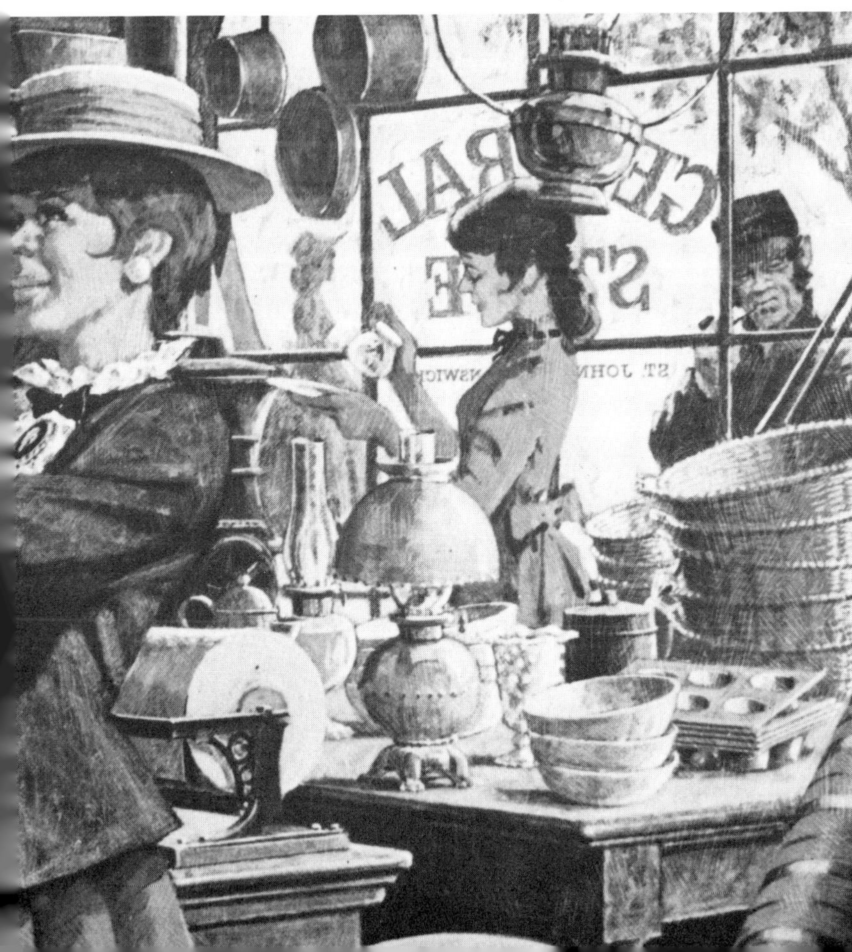

Shastid's friend, Charles F. Prentice, who was a reputable optician, son of British-born optician and instrument maker James Prentice, found himself in a battle royal with ophthalmologist Dr. Henry D. Noyes. Noyes challenged Prentice's right to charge an examining fee in addition to a charge for glasses. Dr. D. B. St. John Roosa, one of Noyes's colleagues, contended that "he [Prentice] must first get a degree of M.D. and then a license to practice. . . ."

It is hard to believe, but when a bill was introduced in the New York State Assembly to regulate the practice of "refracting opticians," opposition came from the ranks of the optometrists themselves. Several urged their fellows to "free yourself from the charge of ancient usages, as the practice that obtained recognition one hundred years ago has been rendered obsolete."

Prentice presented his "Defense of the Optician" at the first hearing on the New York optometry bill in 1896. This impressive document was a milestone in the struggle for the acceptance of opticians. Prentice also gave a demonstration before the Assembly Committee on Public Health in which he used eye models to make his debatable point that adaptation of lenses was "the treating of light and not treating the eye."

In 1908 an optometry law was finally enacted in New York. It established the optometrist's right to examine eyes and prescribe glasses according to certain standards. Optometry laws of some kind now exist in every state and the District of Columbia. But only sixteen states require opticians, who fill prescriptions and fit glasses, to have licenses. Most opticians are trained on the job.

Prentice was a member of the first Board of Examiners established under the New York law. In 1910, he was instrumental in developing a two-year optometry course at Columbia University, which continued until 1956.

After Columbia closed its optometry school, New York was without a college training ground for doctors of optometry (O.D.) until 1971. Because of the acute need for this branch of higher education, the State University became affiliated with the Optometric Center of New York. The Center ceded its research, library, and educational facilities to the University.

The New York State College of Optometry is one of thirteen such institutions in the United States, which graduate eleven hundred students each year. On its staff are ophthalmologists, optometrists, and specialists in basic science, clinical optometry, optometric science, behavioral science, public health, and related subjects. Admission to its four-year professional program requires a minimum of three years of college. The College of Optometry awards a degree in optometry (O.D.) and a graduate degree, Master of Science (M.S.) in Vision Science. In 1976 over five hundred persons applied for the sixty-four available places. The Center is a teaching-clinical institution, so it provides theory and practice simultaneously.

Ophthalmologists object to optometrists' using drugs in eye examinations or as a treatment. This, they contend, is the prerogative of a specialist with an M.D. degree. But in twenty-two states today, optometrists can, after special training, legally use eye drops as anesthetics. Two states have legalized the use of drugs by optometrists for the treatment of certain eye conditions.

Federal laws govern other ophthalmic practices. It is illegal to sell corrective glasses without a prescription. As previously mentioned, all eyeglasses must be of impact-resistant materials. Flammable spectacle frames are outlawed—an important piece of legislation against the use of cellulose nitrate, which is also a component of explosives.

Although the role of optometrists is still not clearly drawn, the approach of some form of national health insurance may serve to clarify the issue. Ophthalmologists and optometrists who are concerned with the welfare of the patient will welcome a resolution of the problem. Both professions deplore the unscrupulous entrepreneur-optometrist, who spends only a few minutes on a so-called eye examination and runs dozens of persons a day through a commercial mill, often prescribing incorrectly and skipping altogether the crucial glaucoma test. The sale of eyeglasses is the name of this game, in which the customer pays too much for too little.

In a nationwide survey, the *Optical Journal and Review of Optometry* reported that 16 percent of the consumers queried didn't know whether they had been examined by an optometrist or an ophthalmologist; 45 percent didn't know the difference between the two. Obviously, the public needs enlightenment.

Continuing Medical Education (CME) now provides credit for ophthalmologists and optometrists who pass examinations on material published in professional periodicals or offered at learning centers. Twenty states now require CME credit for license renewals in several different specialties. Lou Krop, O.D., former president of the New York State Optometric Association, endorses this policy of continuing education and recommends a peer review program for quality control.

Today ophthalmic specialists are showing an increased interest in public health. At the same time the trend in medical care is toward group practice. Many specialists believe solo practice has become too costly. With modern techniques involving expensive diagnostic equipment, a team of several doctors who pool expenses and abilities makes economic sense. Since the public health center will offer the only medical care many persons can afford, the ophthalmologist or optometrist engaged in group practice and devoting part of each week to public health could be the answer for the future.

9

Today and Tomorrow

When French physicist Augustin Jean Fresnel (1788–1827) wrote *Memoir on the Diffraction of Light*, he confirmed Thomas Young's 1802 theory of light. Young had made the first measurements of light wavelengths, and recognized there was a connection between wavelength and the colors of the spectrum. Today, almost two centuries later, the Fresnel findings are considered essential in one of the newest sight aids—press-on optics. These thin, almost weightless, polyvinyl chloride optics will adhere to any lens surface. The vision specialist can experiment with them in varying degrees of lens power or prismatic correction to determine a patient's needs.

The discovery of polymers in this century has caused an explosion of new textiles and other previously nonexistent materials, which are used in such products as vinyl phonograph records, sheet plastics, and these press-on optics. Plastics for eyeglasses, and especially for contact lenses, are rapidly improving. Ocular specialists believe this refinement will eventually make extended-wear contact lenses completely safe.

Electronic techniques will also shape the future of eye care. Some specialists are already using an ophthalmetron, an automatic refracting device. The patient sits passively before this instrument. No subjective reactions are required. When his eyes are measured, his visual acuity is recorded as automatically as the heart's performance is in an electrocardiogram. Automatic refraction has limitations, but it can be done by a doctor's assistant and will probably soon be a part of most eye examinations, especially where large numbers of patients must be tested.

Another device recently introduced is the Humphrey Vision Analyzer, with which refraction is accomplished without the use of a variety of test lenses. The analyzer has a three-foot mirror disk, set several feet in front of the patient, and a console, operated by the examiner. When the patient reports his reaction to the reflected letters, numbers, and symbols on the disk, the examiner enters this information in the machine, which automatically issues a prescription very much as a cash register issues a printed sales total.

It is conceivable that a time will come when an individual can place himself before an ophthalmetron, sit impassively through a test, then move along to a point where, after pushing a button to indicate his preference in frame style, he will receive the spectacles he needs from a vending apparatus. All this will require no human assistance. If the examining instrument finds a vision problem, it will offer a diagnostic print-out that the patient can take to a specialist.

Electronic development has produced a battery of impressive instruments for measurement, analysis, and diagnosis. The electro-retinogram diagnoses ten to fifteen pathological conditions in infants and nonverbal patients. The electro-oculogram records eye movements and detects focusing difficulties. An ultrasonography device views the back of the eye and locates foreign bodies. This device provides the means to detect normal and abnormal tissues when no other visualization is possible. These and other aids are replacing the former educated guesses applied to vision problems.

Ophthalmic surgery is advanced by the binocular microscope and tiny, mechanically controlled instruments guided by the surgeon's foot, which replace the use of the naked eye. These miniaturized techniques have made possible such new operations as vitrectomy to counteract the blinding disease uveitis, which causes cataracts and clouds the eye's iris. By using the Suction Infusion Tissue Extractor (SITE) he developed, Dr. Jay Federman, of Wills Eye Hospital in Philadelphia, extracted the "debris" from the eye of a patient blinded by this disease. Success with this technique, which is not yet perfected, could restore sight in such cases for the first time.

The Russians are experimenting with extensive surgical procedures in ophthalmic correction. In fact, Professor S. M. Fyoderov is quoted in *The Optician,* a professional journal, as saying that the creation of "a new draining system for supplying the optic nerve" can cure glaucoma if done at an early stage. The Russians are developing "a series of operations designed to arrest progressive myopia" in young persons, he reports. Russian specialists even go so far as to predict that eyeglasses may eventually be unnecessary. Surgery may someday be used to change the optical power of the cornea, they say.

This exciting era of progress in many scientific areas holds great promise for the future of eye care and vision aids.

Michel Millodot, of the University of Wales Institute of Science and Technology, reports that blue-eyed persons have corneas twice as sensitive on the average as the corneas of people with brown eyes. Hazel and green-eyed persons fall between these extremes. The study indicates that blue eyes may have more trouble adjusting to contacts. Why is this so? The cornea is a transparent "windshield" over the pupil. Researchers speculate that the corneas of blue-eyed persons contain more nerves. They know that these people react more quickly to drugs. Brown-eyed individuals require stronger dosages for comparable results.

A branch of the science of vision is psychophysics. Those working in this field hope to bridge the gap between the physics of light and the behavior of living organisms by defining with mathematical precision the connection between physical stimuli—lines, points, wavelengths, gradients of texture—and what man sees. This study began in the nineteenth century, when German philosopher Gustav Fechner (1801–1887) developed methods to establish a behavioral unit of measurement.

Photochemistry of the retina, the study of chemical reactions resulting from exposure to light, may ultimately unlock the secrets of the retina, the eye's camera.

It is estimated that there are 350,000 legally blind persons in the United States. In the distant future scientists may reverse the state of blindness in many of them through procedures developed in experiments formerly carried out at the University of Utah Medical Center by biophysicist

William H. Dobelle, computer scientist M. G. Mladejovsky, and others. They were inspired by the 1968 discoveries at the University of London and at Addenbrooke's Hospital, Cambridge, that a blind person could see spots of light called phosphenes when the visual center of the brain was electrically stimulated.

Normally, light sensations reach the visual center in the cerebral cortex at the back of the brain through the optic nerve. Two blind volunteers underwent surgery which temporarily placed sixty-four platinum electrodes against their visual centers. During three days of experiments the volunteers were able to perceive phosphenes in relation to each other. In effect, they saw patterns of light, which appeared as "a constellation of stars."

The hope is that permanent electrode implants in the brain will one day enable a blind person to see objects and to read. Perhaps a glass eye in the eye socket would contain a lens and a subminiaturized camera attached to the eye muscles. (Subminiaturization is a spinoff of the Space Age.) A tiny computer built into an eyeglass frame would translate light into electric current, which would be carried through receivers in the wearer's scalp to the brain implants. However, Dr. Dobelle, who has since transferred his research to the College of Physicians and Surgeons of Columbia University, emphasizes that this prosthesis, even if achieved, would never equal normal sight. And its realization is, at best, many years away.

Blind persons can now receive electronic aid from a device called a Sonicguide. It consists of lightweight eyeglass frames containing an ultrasonic transmitter. The transmitter and two receivers, each about half an inch in diameter, are mounted on the oversized bridge of the eyeglass frame. Inaudible high-frequency sounds are converted into audible signals through the eyeglass temples' electronic circuitry when echoed back from objects within the ultrasonic field. The wearer receives the signals through small, detachable ear tubes from each temple, and carries on a belt or shoulder strap a small control unit with a rechargeable battery. Although it does not replace a cane, the Sonicguide enables the user to avoid contact with unfamiliar objects and to adjust to changing conditions, (e.g., low-hanging, snow-laden tree branches), since he can detect them in advance.

Another device for the blind is the laser cane. When the beams it sends out are interrupted by an obstacle, a buzzer sounds.

Sighted persons are not aware of the acuteness of the other senses, but the blind can substitute touch for sight. Arthur Freese reports that experiments are under way at San Francisco's Smith-Kettlewell Institute of Visual Science to enable the blind to "see" with a TV camera in an eyeglass frame, which picks up impulses and passes them on to over a thousand electrodes in a pad set on the abdomen. The wearer feels the vibrations on his skin in a pattern picked up by the camera.

Blind persons are even now reading printed matter with the aid of an Optacon. This device is also based on the tactile sense. The blind reader receives vibrations against a finger in the shape of a word or letter from light-sensitive phototransistors that scan the print. Optacon users don't read as fast as Braille readers, but their selection is wider, because only a small percentage of published books are translated into Braille or recorded for talking books.

The New York Public Library has recently installed a Kurzweil reading machine that can read the English language in ordinary typeface, produce synthetic speech at 150 words a minute, repeat a passage, and spell the words. According to a report in *The New York Times,* the machine stretches the vowel sounds, making the "voice" speak with a slight accent that is described by some as Swedish.

The future holds promises still undefined. As science uncovers more information about the causes of sight failure, specialists will discover other preventions and cures. Each generation, as in the past, will benefit by this progression. It is unfortunate that many great writers and musicians were born too soon to be saved from painfully poor vision or blindness, among them Milton, Homer, Pepys, Carlyle, Poe, Chopin, De Maupassant. The list is long. One of today's blessings is the certainty that with few exceptions a sighted person, gifted or not, can remain sighted throughout his life.

Conclusion

In *considering* the scientific discoveries of our age, there is always the question—an important one—how will they be used? In eye care the trend is toward public health. Since so many vision problems can be cured if caught early, it is obvious that eye care should be universally available. Dr. Alden Haffner, President of the New York State College of Optometry, believes that the future of eye care will be two-fold. First, he predicts a breakthrough in health services, making them, including eye care, available to all ages and income groups. In other words, he is optimistic about "universal health entitlement." Second, he believes that electronics will unlock many secrets of the visual function, that electronic measurements will establish a relationship between visual development and other phases of development in children. He expects that ocular and brain studies will enable specialists to uncover parallels between the reading process and the achievement process. Dr. Haffner is also hopeful that future tests will reveal the causes of cataracts, which plague the elderly especially, and a way to arrest them.

Such optimism and social awareness is a giant step toward advances on many fronts in the future.

Bibliography

Begbie, G. Hugh, *Seeing and the Eye*. Garden City, N.Y., Natural History Press, 1969.

Brindze, Ruth, *Look How Many People Wear Glasses: The Romance of Lenses*. Paterson, N. J., Atheneum, 1975.

Bronson, L. D., *Early American Specs*. Washington, D.C., Occidental Press, 1974.

Cohen, Neville S. and Joseph L. Shapiro, *Out of Sight into Vision*. New York, Simon & Schuster, 1977.

Corson, Richard, *Fashions in Eyeglasses*. Chester Springs, Pa., Dufour Editions, 1967.

Drew, Ralph, *Professional Ophthalmic Dispensing*. Chicago, Professional Press, 1970.

The Papers of Benjamin Franklin, Vol. 18. Sponsored by the American Philosophical Society and Yale University. New Haven, Connecticut, Yale University Press, 1974.

The Writings of Benjamin Franklin, Vol. 9, 1783–1788. Collected and edited with a Life and Introduction by Albert Henry Smyth. New York, Macmillan, 1906.

Freese, Arthur, *The Miracle of Vision*. New York, Harper & Row, 1977.

Karlins, Marvin, and Lewis M. Andrews, *Biofeedback: Turning on the Power of Your Mind*. Philadelphia, Lippincott, 1972.

McDonald, Linda, *Contact Lenses: How to Wear Them Successfully*. New York, Doubleday, 1972.

"Optometry, The Profession. Its Antecedents, Birth and Development." A series of editorial articles from *The Optical Journal and Review of Optometry* (October 1, 1945–January 1, 1947).

Rudolph, Mae, and Conrad Mueller, *Light and Vision*. New York, Time-Life, 1966.

Solomon, Herbert and Walter J. Zinn, *The Complete Guide to Eye Care, Eyeglasses and Contact Lenses*. New York, Frederick Fell, 1977.

Young, Patrick, "Cataract Counterattack." *The National Observer* (May 22, 1976).

Index

Kelley, Alberta

Lenses, spectacles, eyeglasses, and contacts

DATE			